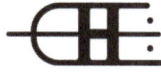

Holistic Collaboration Series Presents Book #2

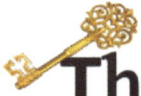

The Movement Connection

An Adaptable Exercise Routine for Flexibility and Strengthening

Body and Soul Nutrition

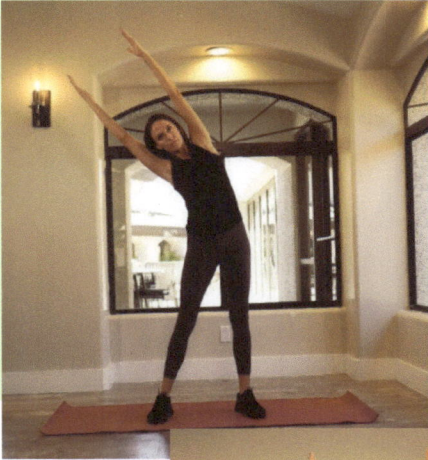

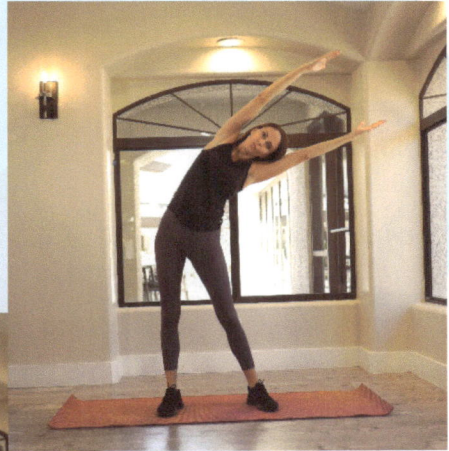

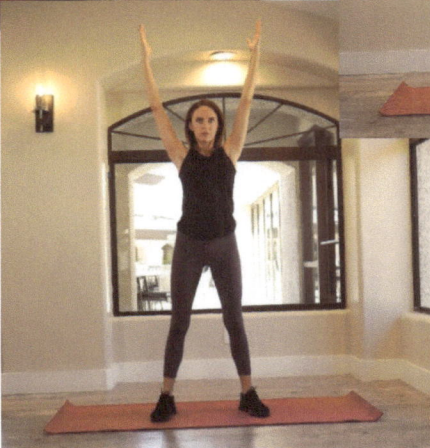

By Sherry Bainbridge PhD
Model: Jennifer Cole

Holistic Collaboration Series:
The Movement Connection – Body and Soul Nutrition
By, Sherry Bainbridge PhD

ISBN: Print – 978-1-7358688-0-6
ISBN: Ebook – 978-1-7358688-1-3

https://holisticcollaboration.com
Previous Publications: Connecting Poetry -
Body and Soul Nutrition (2019)
YouTube: Peeves, Tips, and Tricks
TikTok: Sherry's Snippets

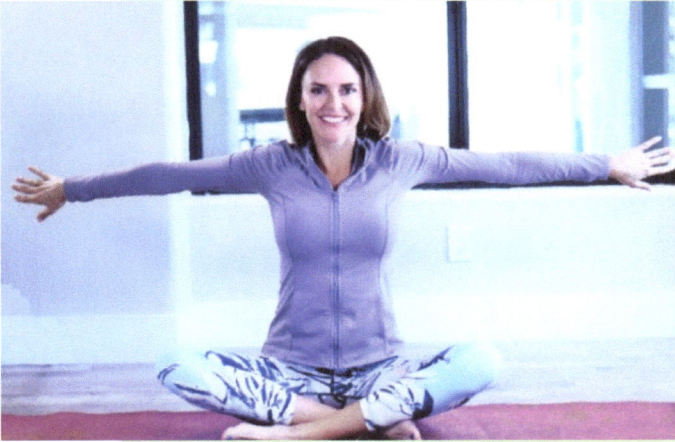

Moving Is The Best!

Disclaimer:

Never stop taking your medications without your professional licensed medical teams' input. Please inform them of any changes in life-style. Their access to information and technology can be most helpful in tracking and validating your health and well-being efforts. Nothing in this book is a replacement for a professional licensed mental and physical health consultation, evaluation, or treatment. You are worth it! Know limitations, care for and listen to the body, the mind, and the heart. Please, seek advice and guidance when it is needed.

Contents

Introduction

The Movement Connection is an exercise routine for physical activity, toning, and improving the relationship with the body and the spirit. These 44 exercises and stretches help the body with increasing movement, flexibility, strength, and balance. They are adaptable to almost any body type, including those with injuries or are pregnant. The routines design helps with the safety of the neck, lower back, lower abdomen, shoulders, and joints. Many have contributed to the routine's development. As with all things, we simply cannot do anything without the help of other people!

I like doing a memorized routine. It takes away excuses. No gym, no special equipment, all that is needed is the right mindset, a little clean floor space, and something to help with balance like a chair.   Intentional exercise aids body oxygen, mood balancing, getting rid of toxins, eliminations, improved circulation, tightening the skin, increasing energy, pain management (1), aiding in sleep, the list goes on (2). Exercise has too many benefits to ignore. Give this routine a try and let me know how this has worked for you and what you did to make it work? Thank you very much. Collaborating helps everyone.

Be sure to be comfortable, hydrated, appropriately dressed, and in a safe environment.

Always be aware of where every part of the body is at all times. This approach is a form of being present. It is particularly important to those with challenges. Do each exercise correctly and with excellent posture.

Safety is of the utmost importance. Learn your boundaries well, and be very careful when working with chronic pain. Discomfort is okay; pain is not! Stop before it gets worse, back off, relax, breathe, and for now, move on and try later. If needed, seek professional physical therapy assistance to ensure all exercises are accurately adjusted to accommodate any injuries or limitations.

The routine is also an opportunity to listen to how and what the energy body and physical body communicate. Emotion, sensations, and thoughts all contribute to physical and energetic/spiritual communications. Stop thinking, see and feel yourself heathy. Allow the Divine to give guidance the way it has for already an eternity. We and others get inside our heads too much. Exercise is an opportunity to clear thought, focus on a dream, and re-establish spirit connection. It aligns the mind, body, and spirit. Aligning causes energy to step up and aid us in our life visions.

The world uses repetition to influence how a person feels and thinks. Science has proven that repetition rewires the brain. So why not use this to our advantage? See yourself connecting with your amazing body. Feel how great it feels to consistently exercise. Align the dream with internal and external energy through feeling it. See it. This is what leads to physical manifestation. Be honest, no expectations, just do your part. No discussion needed. **Moving is a must.**

Emotion, is where the greatest power rests. Choose your emotions. Decide now to get excited about moving the body. See how great the skin looks, balance increases, and confidence rises.
It is an attitude, a choice, a decision that this is amazing and fun. Just plaster a smile on the face, the energy body immediately changes. A most powerful tool when used appropriately.

Being in motion is a gift, a pleasure, and is a tremendous aid to overall well-being. With so many rewards, prioritizing exercise is a must. When we step up, it is a chance to build discipline, heal, and boosts confidence. Doing is motivating, so stop thinking and just do.

This routine flows smoothly from one exercise to the other. It makes it easy to meditate and motivate. The *asterisks* and tips are about what others and myself may concentrate on while doing the routine. Become incompatible with thoughts and actions that are not loving, kind, honest, and supportive.

The Movement Connection starts with the exercises sitting on the floor, then laying, and then standing. 10-20+ repetitions are a good goal for most. Do what you can and work up to those that are more difficult by increasing them 2 - 5 each week until you can do the desired repetitions.

Each exercise is to be done slowly and unrushed, with proper form and posture. A mirror or two can be a great way to check the appropriate form. If there are injuries or limitations to consider, seek professional therapy to determine how to alter exercises correctly.

The last exercise in the Movement Connection is a meditative and connecting stance used in Qi Gong. It is physically and spiritually healing, energizing, grounding, and balancing. ***My most favorite!***

Emotionally and physically supporting the body is an art. It is creative, nurturing, and fun if you choose to think of it this way. By stepping up to ourselves, we encourage healing, learning, improved connections with others, and the environment. "The physical body and the emotional body will support the physical and emotional plate we feed it every single time."

Never exaggerate or lie with your body. Be gentle, kind, patient, and honest. The body knows if its caretaker is listening and healthfully acting. It will then begin to communicate more clearly. Give yourself a hug, smile, and show the body it can depend on you.

Pema Chodron titled one of her books: "Start Where You Are." Let go of the rest! Let's get connected, get moving, and keep moving. Do not give up! We are ultimately one and affected by what each other thinks and does. We depend on and need each other! Following is an at-a-glance list for quick referencing. ***Make it fun!***

Tips: When you feel resistant, change your thinking, environment, something to alter things. You really do have more influence than you realize.

(1) Guy L McCormack, Pain Management by Occupational Therapists. American Journal of Occupational Therapy, September 1, 1988, Updated April 30, 2020. Vol. 42, 582-590. https://doi.org/10.5014/ajot.42.9.582

(2) Jerath, R., Crawford, M.W., Barnes, V.A. et al. Self-Regulation of Breathing as a Primary Treatment for Anxiety. Appl Psychophysiol Biofeedback 40, 107–115 (2015). https://doi.org/10.1007/s10484-015-9279-8 Published April, 14, 2015

The Movement Connection At-A-Glance Exercise List:

Sitting on Floor Section – starts on page 14:

1. **Rhythmic Breathing:** Breathe in, hold, exhale, and hold

2. **Neck and Spine Stretch:** Chin to ceiling/chest, roll down/up

3. **Shoulder Lift:** Arms above head, lift shoulders up and down.

4. **Side Stretch:** Ear toward shoulder, chin the wall

5. **Range of Motion Neck Stretch:** Face side to side

6. **Forward/Back Neck Stretch:** Head forward/backwards

7. **Shoulder Blade, palms facing:** Forwards/backwards

8. **Shoulder Blade, palms facing chest:** Forward/backwards

9. **Spinal Roll:** Chin to chest, roll down and up

10. **Side Arm Stretch:** Fingers up, palms towards wall

11. **Shoulder Rolls:** Large circles forwards and backwards

12. **Arm and Elbow Stretch:** Arm above head, hand on back

13. **Sitting Waist Twist:** Turn waist, look over shoulder

14. **Prayer Strengthening:** Prayer hand and arm series

15. **Sitting Side Stretch:** One leg bent, other to side

16. **Side Leg Lift:** One leg bent, one to side, lift/lower

17. **Front Leg Lift:** One leg bent, one straight in front, lift/lower.

18. **Eagle Spread Stretch:** Spread both legs to side

Laying Down on Floor – starts on page 35:

19. **Body Stretch:** On back, arms above head

20. **Curl Up:** Bring knees to the chest

21. **Pelvic Tilt:** Spine flat, raise/lower pelvic

22. **Ankle/Foot Point Flex and Strengthen:** Point and flex

23. **Lower Back and Abdomen Stretch:** Bend leg, cross it over the other knee

24. **Straight-Back Sit-ups:** Hands crossed in front

25. **Sit-ups for Lower Abdomen:** Hands behind the head

26. **Side Leg Stretch:** Lift leg, bend toward chest, straighten, side, up, and down

27. **Knee and Leg Raises:** Leg behind, stretch, to chest

28. **Cat Stretch:** Roll towards ceiling, then arch

29. **Doggie Leg Lift:** Lift one bent leg then the other

30. **Push-ups:** Nose to ground then away from ground

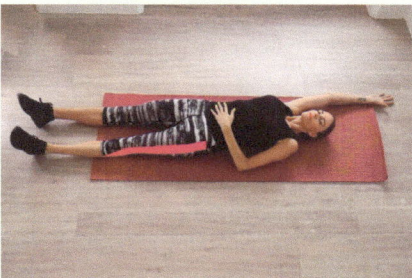

It is a gift to move the body.

The Movement Connection At-A-Glance Exercise List Continued:

Standing – starts on page 47:

31. **Stand Up and Stand Tall:** Stretch tall

32. **Standing Side Stretch:** Arms up, face forward, bend waist

33. **Ridding Negative Energy:** Throw out negative energy

34. **Stirring in Positive Energy:** Take in positive energy

Feeling Awesome!

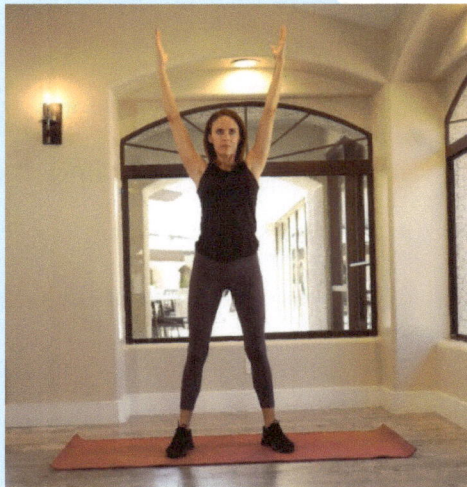

Chair – starts on page 50:

35. **Horse Stance:** Hold chair back, sit down into stance

36. **Calf Lift:** Bend knee to lift calf up/down

37. **Side Chair Calf Lift:** Lift calf up/down

38. **Side Chair Leg and Hip Stretch:**
    Heel to floor, sit into it

39. **Plantar Fasciitis Stretch:** Balance on balls of feet

40. **Lunge with Straight Leg:**
    Next to chair, lung forward

41. **Sitting Leg and Knee Stretches:**
    Hand presses on knee

42. **Knee Circles:** Bend knee, lift leg, do large calf circles

43. **Sitting Knee and Thigh Stretch:**
    Hand guides knee to side

44. **The Wuji:** Stand like a tree and get connected.

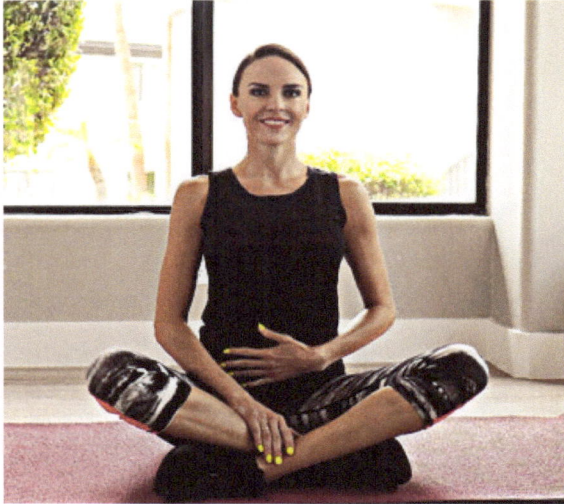

1. Rhythmic Breathing

Sit comfortably with legs crossed, good posture and a smile: Back is lined up, neck is tall, chin slightly down, shoulders relaxed (slightly dropped, kept down, straight, and centered with the torso (do not raise the shoulders). The pelvic is slightly tucked under and forward. All should be comfortable and pain-free. Experience the nice gentle stretch.

*Now, steadily breathe in the breath of the divine. The energy of the creator, the beginning of life. Visualize and intend balancing and healing for the mind, body, and energy. Let the Divine healing white light of grace and love travel down through the crown (top, middle of the head) of the head. Have the brilliant light cleanse and calm as it goes down through the center of the torso. It is relaxing the body further as it passes through the pelvic, the legs and the feet. Safely connecting with Creation and Mother Earth.

This is a type of grounding. It sets the stage for Divine guidance and knowledge. We take in and release energy vibrations that contain information and influence future events.

*Air is God's breath both in and out. When air comes in, it cleans, grounds, balances, gathering up anything negative, noticing and riding sabotages or blockages. (I like placing all these in a balloon and safely blowing it up-BOOM.) When you take a breath in, hold it for a few seconds, then gently release it to safely carry out and dissolve what is not supporting your healthy goals. When breathing in, replace the energy with peaceful healing love. Do not want to have vulnerable holes left in the energy body. While properly breathing (see below), try to create moments with no thought.

*Try to see through the mind's eye (gently close your eyes and look toward the center top of the nose, about a 1/2 inch down), your very own spark of the divine can be seen here. Give it time. It may be minimal, but it is there, it is bright and radiant white. When recognized, feel it, intend it to grow. Doesn't matter if it does or not. Connect with the energies of its pure love, strength, and wisdom. These loving vibrations and frequencies are calming and balancing to the disruptive waves.

Every organ and system have its unique healthy vibration. Energy is intelligent and when directed for healing, it seeks to balance. They are attracted. However, when pulsating energy waves are out-of-whack; they will draw in similar chaotic or low energy frequencies that can lead to more severe life situations and health issues. The body is speaking-up by making things worse so it can be noticed. If we are listening, we can choose otherwise before inviting in a health crisis. This is why energy and touch therapies are supportive and effective.

You Got This!

To properly breathe; use the lower abdomen like a baby does. It should expand first, then the chest. While exhaling, the abdomen lowers first, followed by the chest. Try to do his throughout the day.

Rhythmic/abdominal breathing begins with holding the inhaled breath a moment or two then exhaling. At the end of the exhale, hold it a moment or two, then repeat breathing in, holding, exhaling, hold… Repeat 3-5 times.

Studies show that this technique when combined with visualizing (using the imagination to create scenes and stories) helps with relaxation, releases physical and mental stress (1), and reduces chronic pain (2). These techniques put the mind, the body, and the energy system on the same page towards a goal. **Our goal here is to keep the body moving!**

Tips: When doing the more strenuous part of an exercise, gently and steadily breathe out; the less strenuous; gently and steadily breathe in.

**The body has its own brain.
It knows only what you have taught it!**

Smile and feel happiness flood through the body and spirit. *Simple right?*

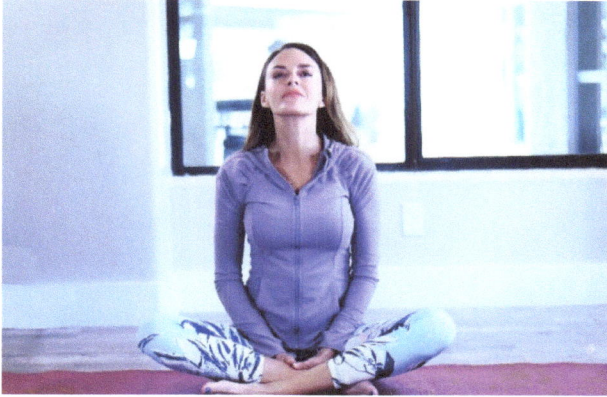

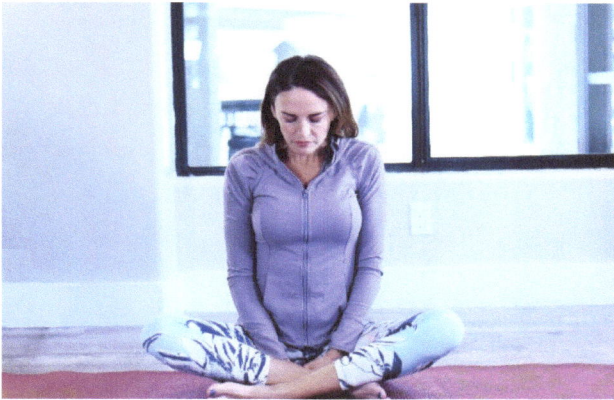

2. Neck and Spine Stretch

Sit straight, head square with the shoulders, gently move chin toward the ceiling, stretching the front of the neck. Make sure to keep the shoulders down and centered while keeping the back straight.

Move the chin towards the chest, stretching the back of the neck and spine, which will also pull and stretch the shoulder blade muscles. Continue to breathe in and out to make sure there is a steady flow of oxygen. Hold the stretch 15-30 seconds.

*Sometimes I visualize little army men going up and down with ropes to clear out and clean out my veins. **Make it fun!**

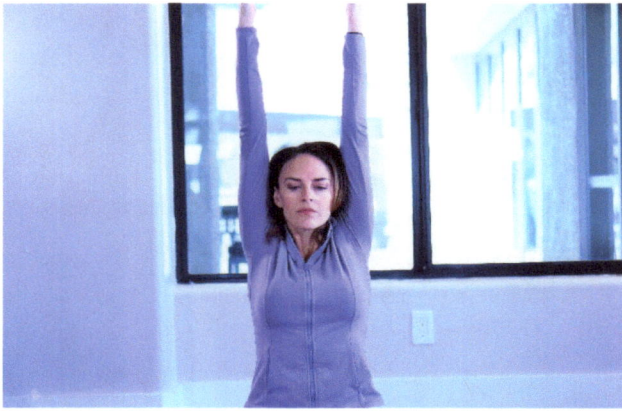

3. Shoulder Lift

Arms stretched above the head with palms facing each other; pull shoulders straight up and down. The palms should not move toward each other. Pull up and down with the shoulders only. Inhale when pulling up and exhale when pulling down. Arms are kept straight. The Shoulder Lift is a very isolated movement.

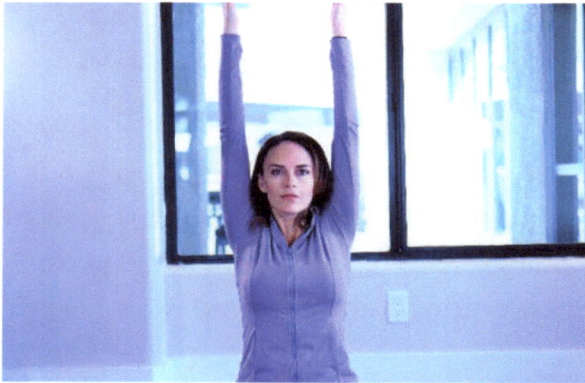

*Mantras are another one I like to do. I stay away from those that focused on material or monetary gain.

There are many different mantras. The Deities are just a form of focus. My experience has shown that statues and other idols often have unwanted attached beings. I limit how many I have around and do intentional cleansing for those I do.

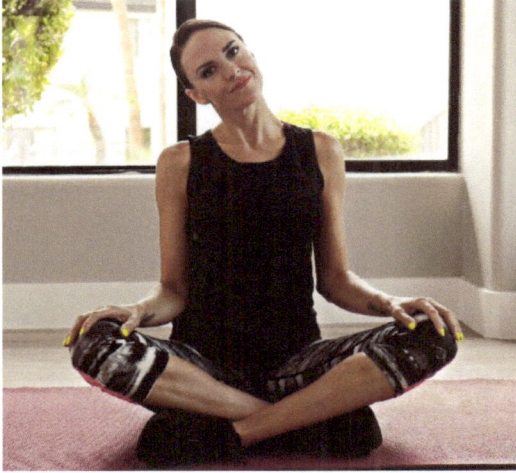

4. Neck Side Stretch

Head should be squarely over the shoulders. Keep the spine straight, and keep the shoulders down and even. Move the ear towards one shoulder and the chin towards the wall stretching the neck, and hold the stretch for 15-30 seconds.

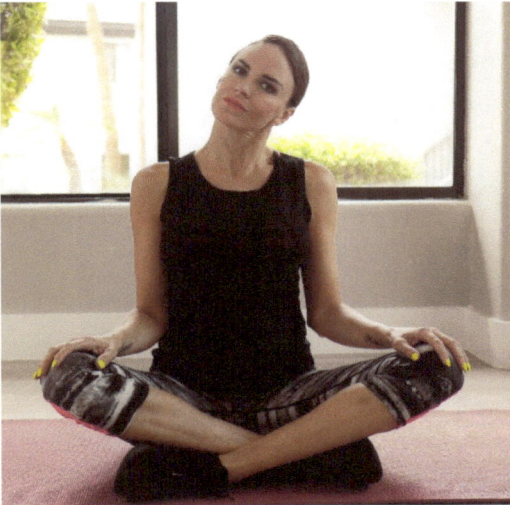

Do the same number of stretches for each side. Do 5-10 sets. These stretches are very good for aiding in relieving pain.

Resistance is when our body is feeling our thinking. Usually about historical experiences – get out of the past. **This is now!**

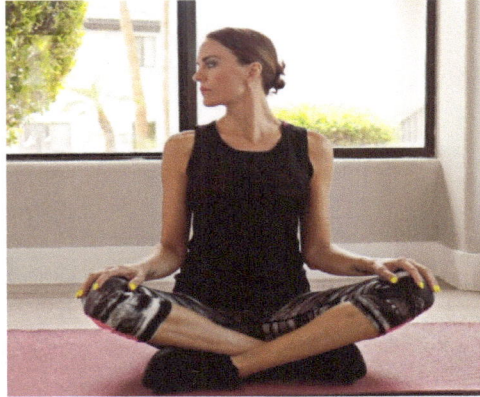

5. Range of Motion Neck Stretch

Keep head square to the shoulders and the shoulders level and kept down. Look to one side, use the forefinger to help stretch the neck just a touch more. Hold the stretch 15-30 seconds. Gently do one side then the other. Do 10 sets.

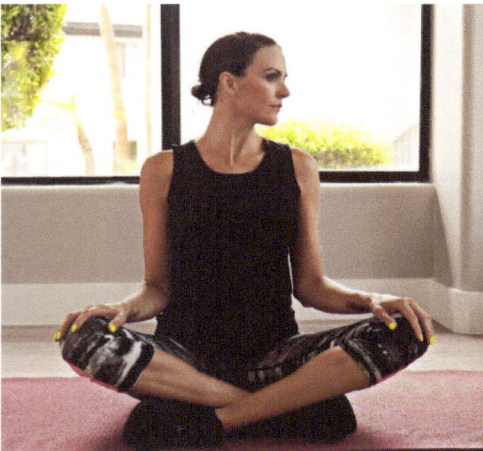

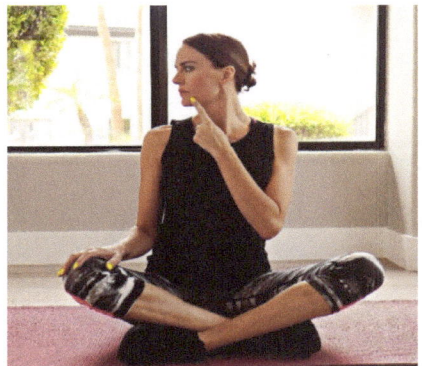

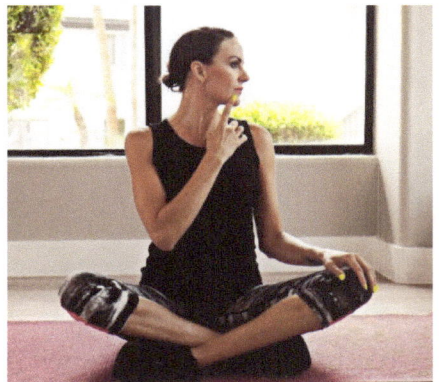

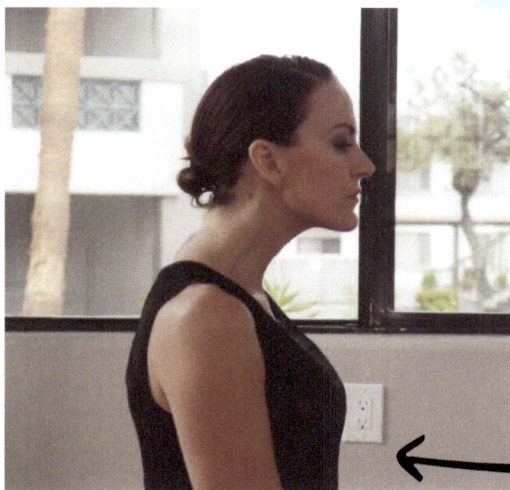

The real turtle-neck.

6. Forward/Back Neck Stretch

Keep the head square to the shoulders, and shoulders level and kept down. Like a turtle, move the face forward then back. This exercise is great to do at a desk, in the bathroom, or in the car.

This exercise helps avoid that upper hump forming at the base of the neck and spine.

Not the most attractive exercise but very effective.

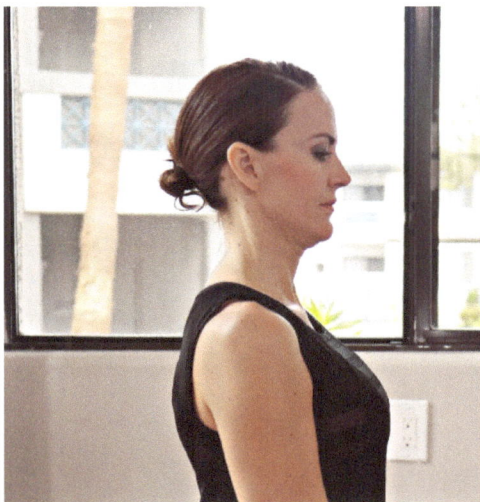

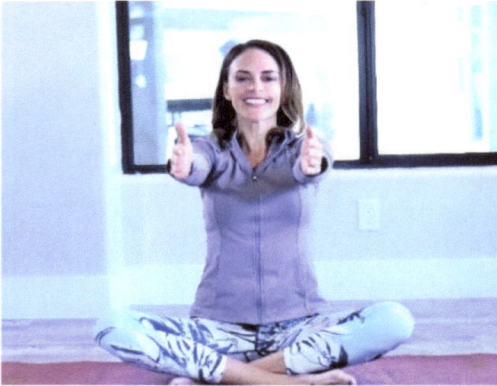

7. Shoulder Blade Stretch, Palms Facing

Arms outstretched in front, shoulder-width, palms facing. Keep shoulders down. The shoulders go straight back, pulling the shoulder blades together, then move forward, pulling the shoulder blades apart. These are slow and fluid motions. Keep shoulders level.

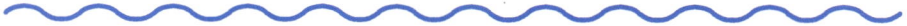

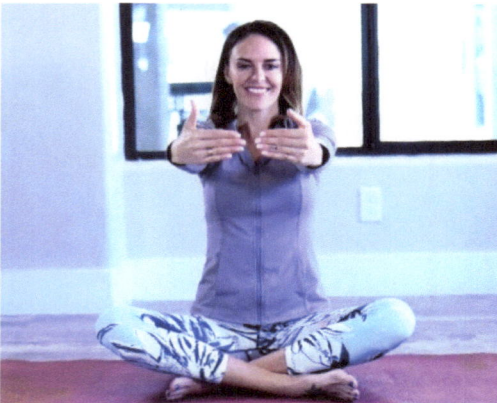

8. Shoulder Blade Stretch Palms Facing Chest

Face the palms towards the chest, and again, move the arms forward, separating shoulder blades, then move the arms back, bringing the shoulder blades together.

9. Spinal Roll

Gently place hands on the top back of the head.

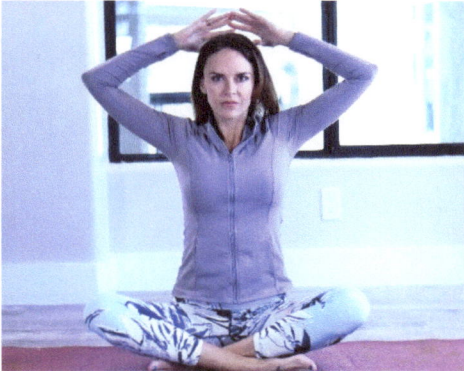

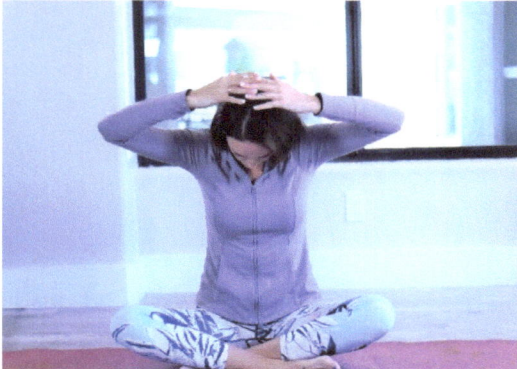

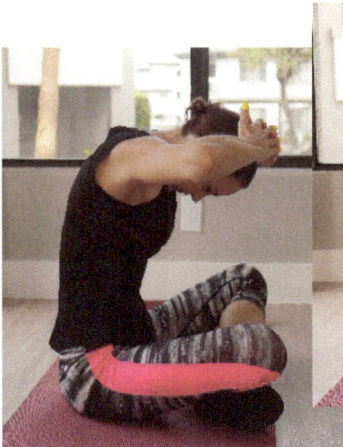

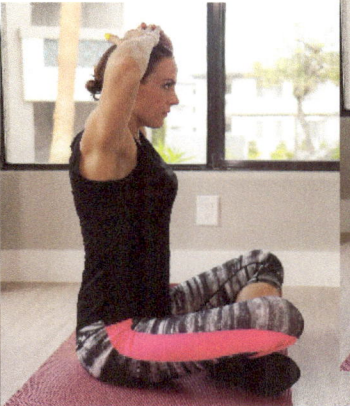

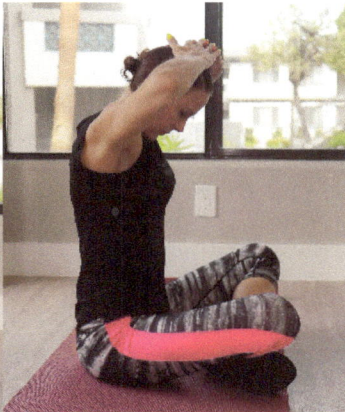

Slowly roll downward, one vertebra after another going as low as is comfortable. Let the back bending naturally by rolling head towards the abdomen.

Stop and hold the stretch a bit before moving lower.

Be kind and go safely as low as you can. In time it will become easier to go lower.

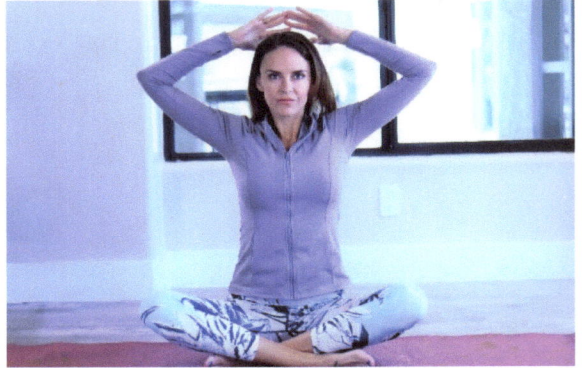

Unroll up one vertebra at a time until you have once again returned to the starting position. Neck and spine strength and flexibility play a huge roll in our balance.

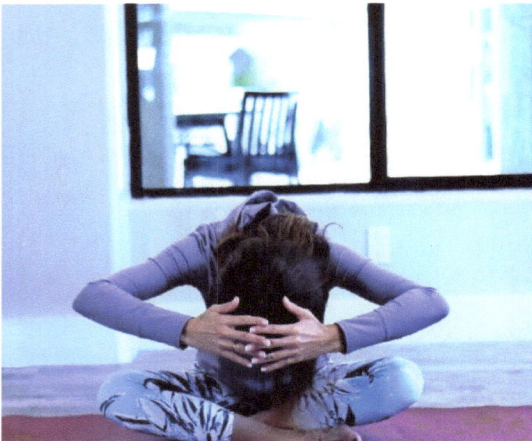

Tips: Be very careful with spinal injuries. It is wise to check with a professional so that you are clear on any needed adaptations. The spine includes the head, neck, and backbone. Its care and health influence the immune system.

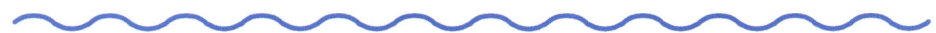

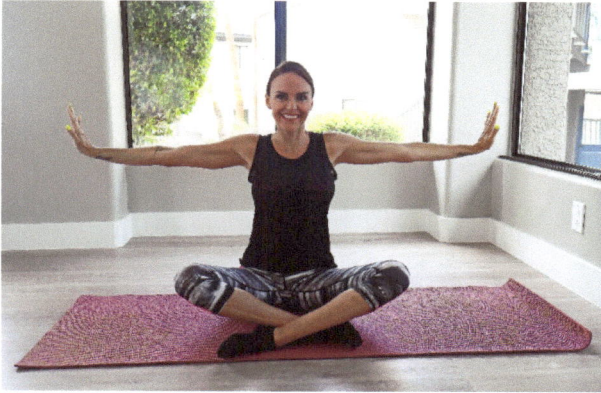

10. Side Arm Stretch, Fingers Up

Shoulders down and centered, arms out-stretched and level with the shoulders, palms facing the walls, and the fingers are pointing towards the ceiling. While holding arms out, relax the fingers, hands, and elbows to rest a moment. Then repeat pressing palms toward walls. It is normal to feel tingling in the fingers and hands when doing this one.

11. Shoulder Rolls

Move each shoulder in a big circular motion backward and then forwards. Try not to move other parts of the body. Keep this very specific to each shoulder.

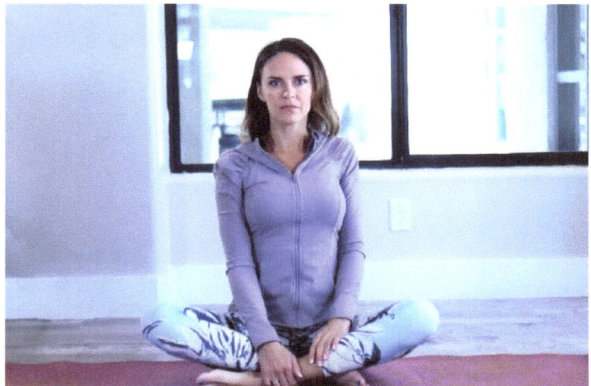

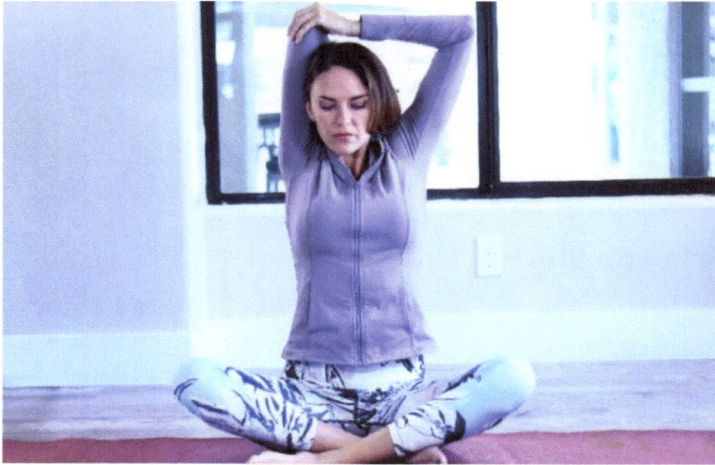

12. Arm and Elbow Stretch

Lay hand flat against the muscle between the spine and shoulder blade and stretch the underarm from elbow to keep the arm straight, as shown in the picture here. Gently press the elbow to increase the stretch. Hold for 15-30 seconds.

13. Sitting Waist Twist

Turn to stretch the waste by looking behind. Stretch one side then the other. Great for balance and flexibility.

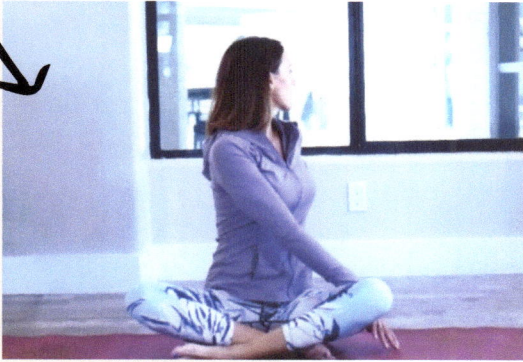

Nice twist Jennifer.

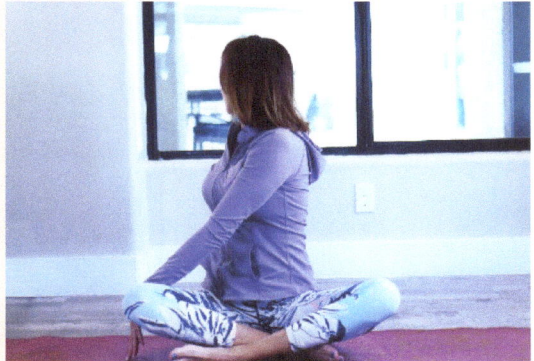

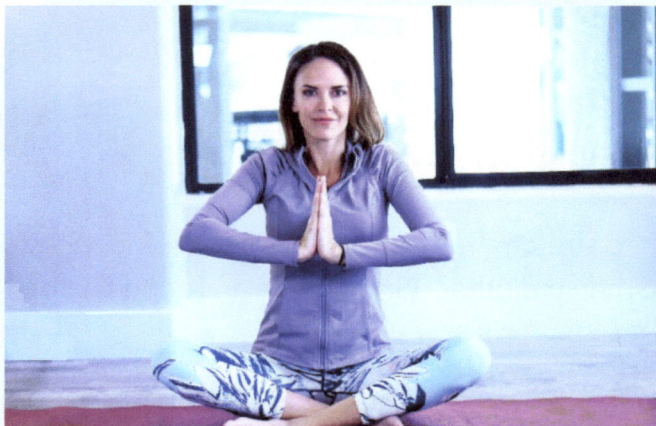

14. Prayer Strengthening

Keep shoulders down, press palms together, and keep pressing with a little pressure. Ease the forearms together along with comfortable pressure. Go back down into the prayer position.

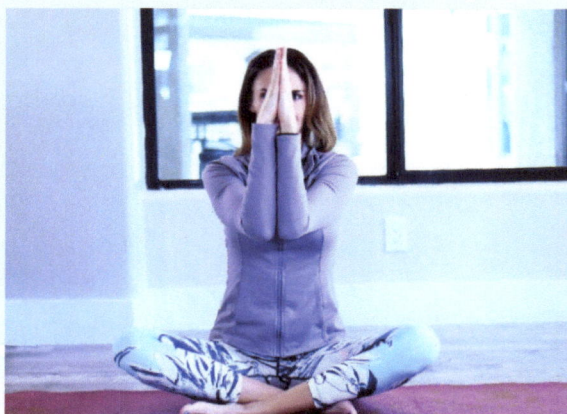

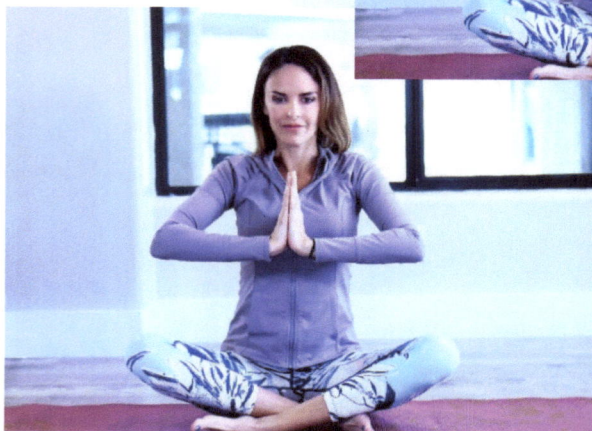

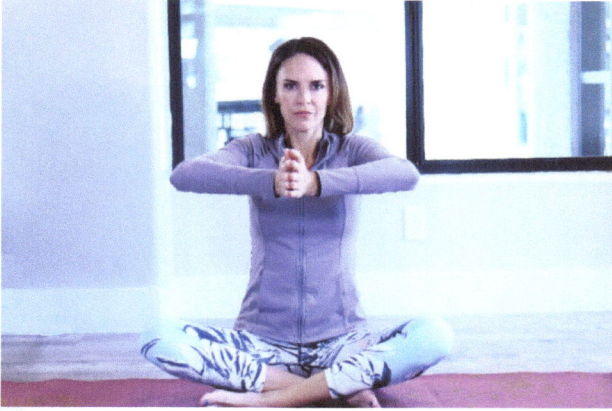

Turn the fingers and point them forward, still pressing the hands together. Shoulders and elbows lined up and centered. Hold this 15-30 second

Slowly straighten the arms in front with palms still together.

Turn palms outward.

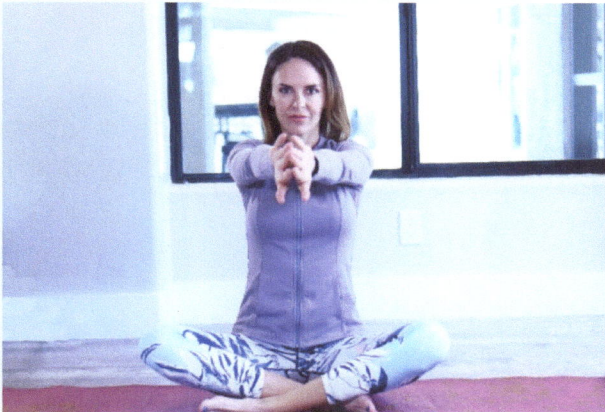

Just like dancing – fun!

I love to move my body!

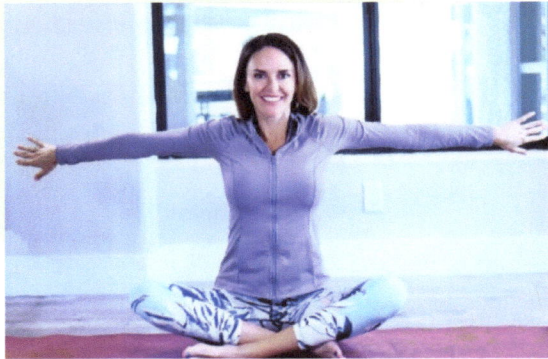

Then turn palms forward and bring arms back together in front with palms facing each other, continue a bit of pressure.

As if pulling the palms and arms through the water. Keep even with shoulders and stretch the arms as back as they can go comfortably into a T.

Ending in the prayer position.

Pull the arms around to line up with them aligned the shoulders.

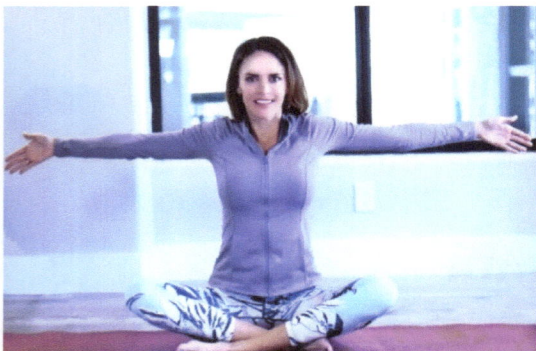

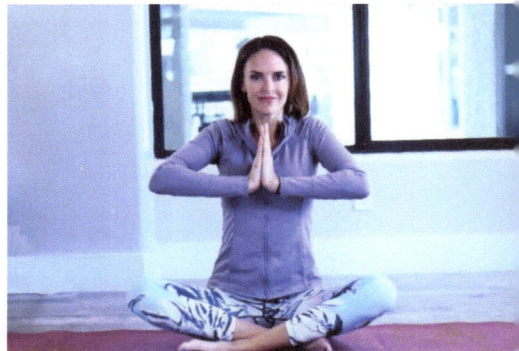

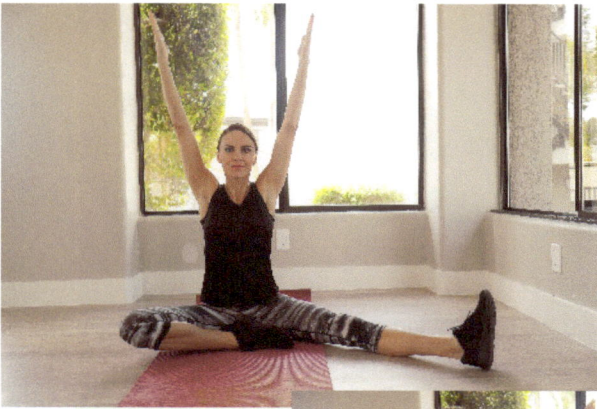

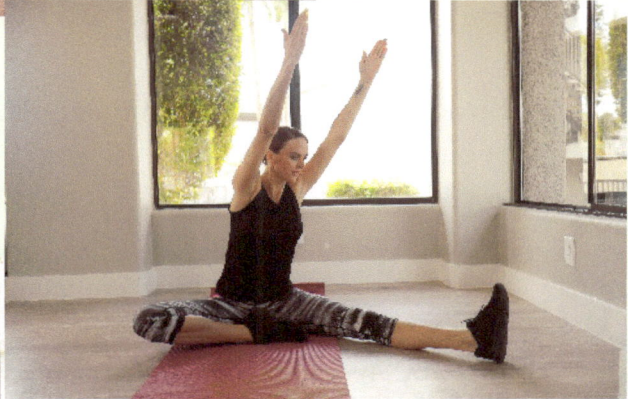

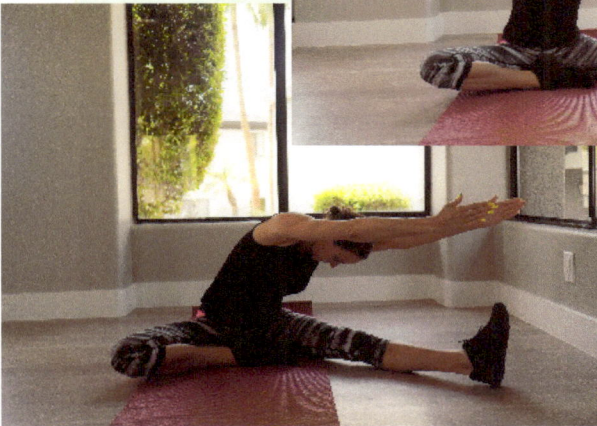

15. Sitting Side Stretch

Make sure pelvic is flat on the floor. Put one leg stretched to the side and bend the other knee as shown. Sit with spine straight and tall. Flex the foot for added stretch. Arms stretched upwards with palms facing, turn torso towards the out-stretched leg and bend the chest towards the knee. Inhale as you raise the body and exhale as you lower the body.

16. Side Leg Lift

From the same position as in #14, pull the stomach against the spine. Lengthen the entire leg, pushing the heel toward the wall. For balance hold, onto the ankle and calf of the bent leg. Do not lift buttock's cheek and keep the foot flexed. Try to keep the spine straight. Gently lift the outstretched leg a couple of inches off the ground as you exhale. Hold a few seconds, then relax the leg and inhale. Repeat

This can be a tough exercise for some people. Keep trying. It will happen. After this exercise, shake the legs out to help relax the muscles.

Tips: As the body strengthens, try not to lower leg all the way to the floor. Gently lift and lower keeping leg off the ground.

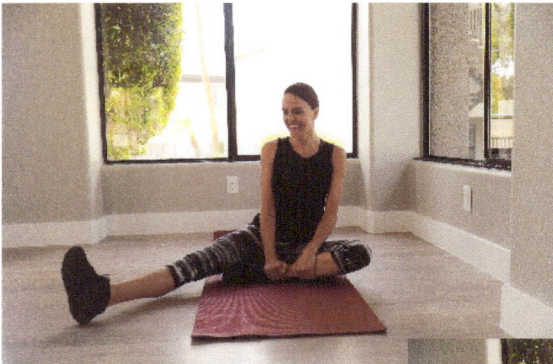

(Jennifer is cracking up at how hard these are-LOL)

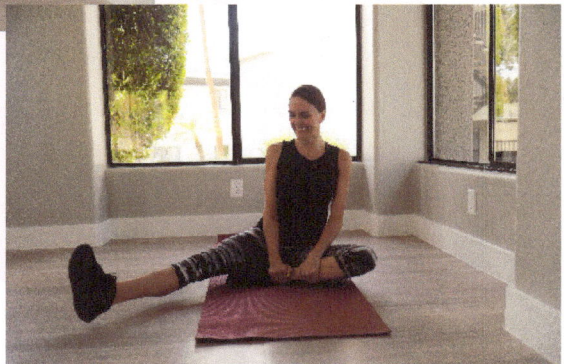

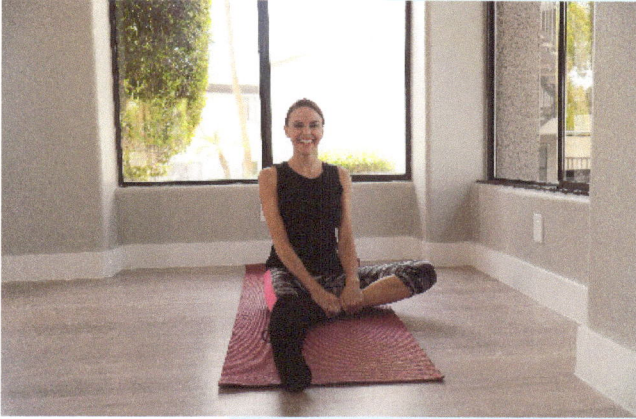

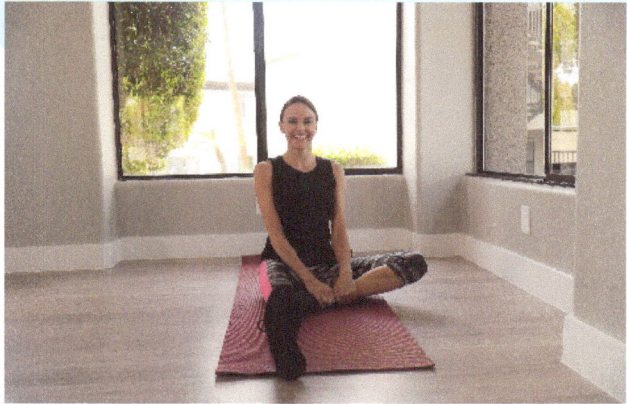

17. Front Leg Lift

Now place the outstretched leg in front and the foot flexed, pointing the toes towards the body. Round the back slightly. Lift leg a couple of inches. Hold, then relax the leg. As with #15, it can be altered to increase strength by not relaxing the leg in between movements. Gently lift then lower and repeat. Exhale during lift.

The body is our very own baby to care for.

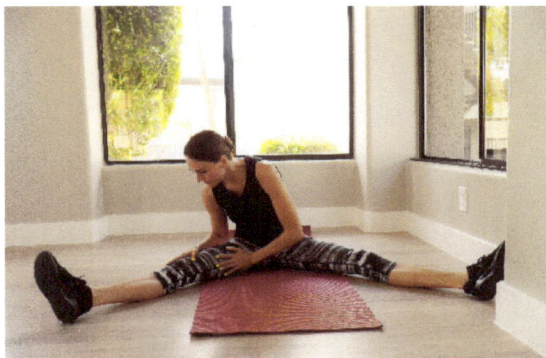

18. Eagle Spread Stretch

Stretch both legs out in front and as wide as is comfortable. Tighten the buttocks and flatten the stomach. Ensure the pelvis in flat on the floor (means that there is no arch in the lower back). Gently turn torso toward the outstretched leg and move head and chest towards the knee. Try not to bend the back. Keep feet flexed, and stay relaxed. Do not push too much, stop and hold for a of moments, then sit up. Repeat with the center and the other leg.

〜〜〜〜〜〜〜〜〜〜〜〜

Tips: Be careful not to stretch too hard. Do not want to tearing the inner thigh muscle. If muscles are tight, rub them with the palms. It is helpful to massage and warm the muscles.

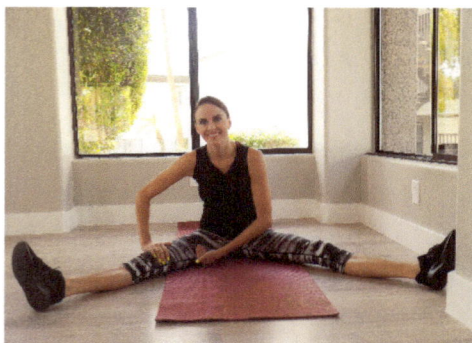

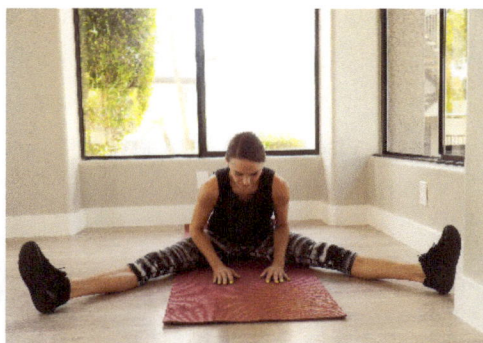

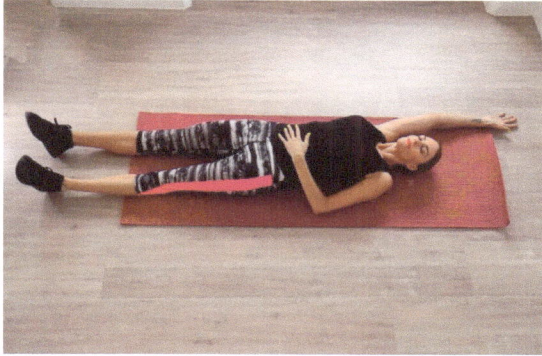

19. Laying Down Body Stretch

Flatten the entire spine against the mat.   Reach one arm at a time above the head and stretch from head to toe, then relax, and repeat. Take a few good deep breaths.

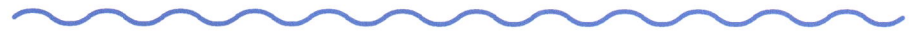

~~~~~~~~~~~~~~~~~~~~~~~~~~~~~~~~~

Tips: Intend chakras to spin at the correct speed, in the right direction, at the accurate size, in perfect harmony with itself, energy, mind, and body.

20. Curl Up

Bring knees up to the chest, place hands on the ankles and stretch the lower back as the hands press the legs and knees towards the floor. Lighten the hold and relax, repeat.

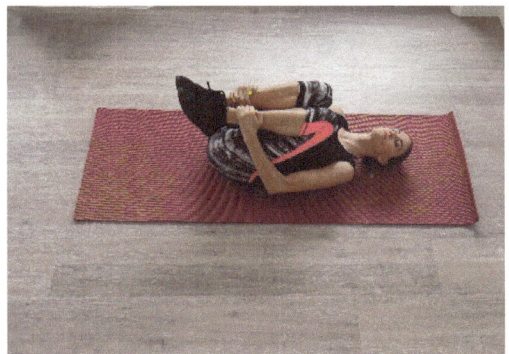

21. Pelvic Tilt

Lay on the back and bend the knees. Place hands palm side down, under the lower back and upper buttock's cheek to aid in supporting the lower back and stomach muscles. Gently lift the pelvis upwards and then slightly roll the lower back and pelvis back onto the hands, repeat.

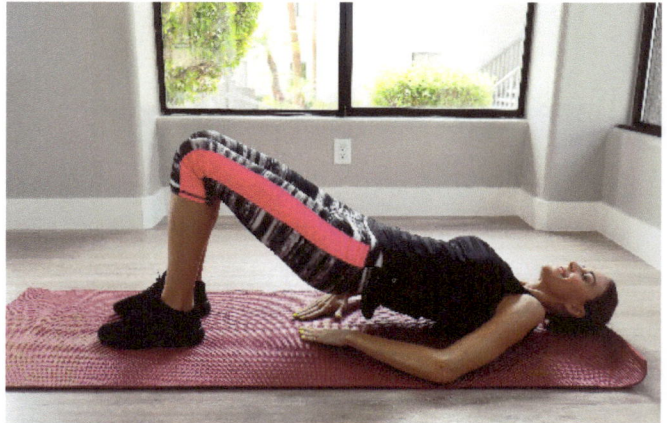

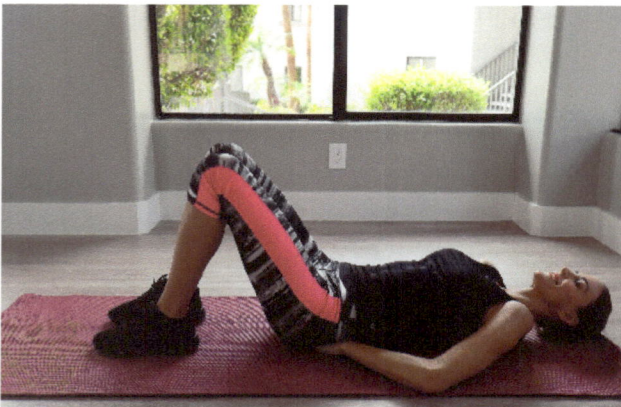

My intention today is to use kind words towards myself!

*Great time to also work with the energy body. Picture your aura, see or imagine the chakras. Say the following:

"All chakras spin at the appropriate size, in the correct direction, and at the right speed. In perfect harmony with all the energy system and the physical body."

Change is uncomfortable. Tell the body to help and not to draw you back. I got this!

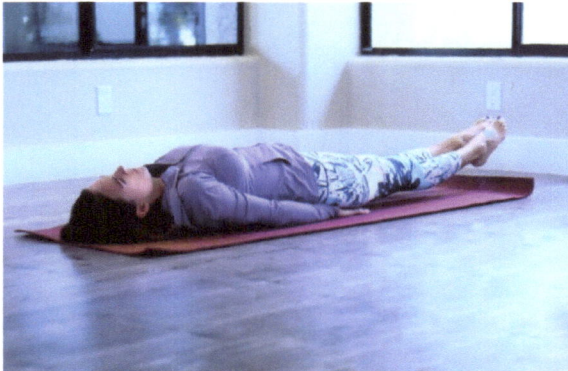

22. Ankle and Feet Point, Flex, and Strengthen

Exhale, pull the stomach in and press the waist on the mat. Place hands underside of buttocks cheek. Flex the feet, bringing the toes towards the body, lift both legs a few inches off the ground and hold, then point toes towards the wall and hold. Relax legs against the mat and repeat. This exercise will strengthen the abdomen and help the spine more limber. Shake out arms and legs.

23. Lower Back and Abdomen Stretch

Lay flat on the floor. Outstretch the arms, relax the neck, press the lower back and stomach against the floor. Lay straight and tall yet relaxed. Lift one leg at a time, bend the knee in an "L" shape. Place the opposite hand on the knee as you carefully cross the other leg. Gently press the knee and leg down to stretch the lower back. Repeat

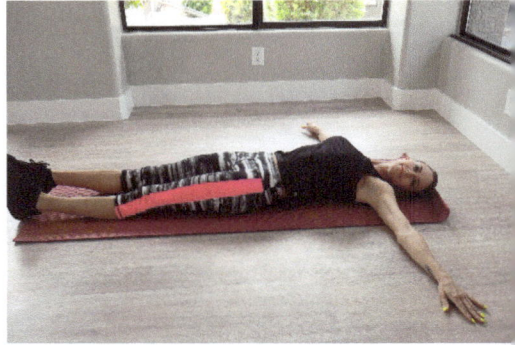

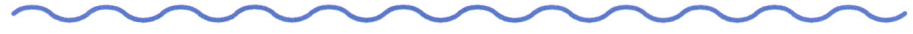

Tip: Great to do every day! Stretches and straightens lower spine, muscles, and increases blood flow.

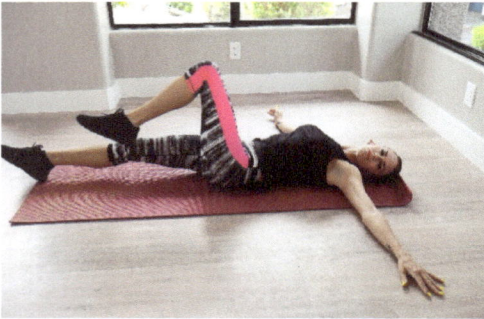

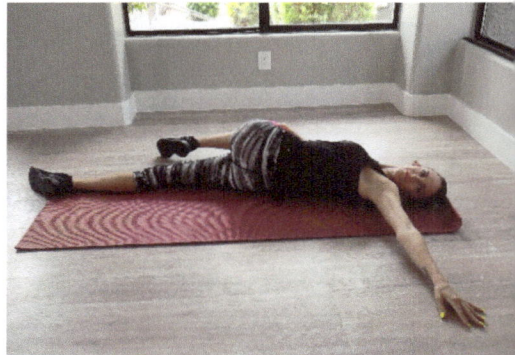

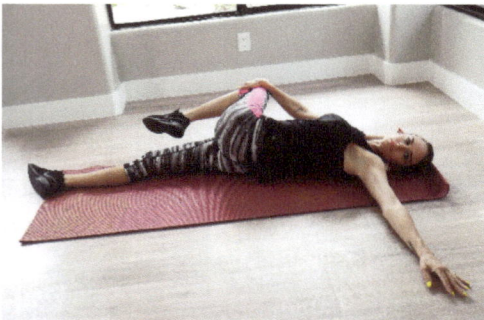

24. Straight-Back Sit-ups for All the Abdomen

Cross hands over the chest to aid the lower abdomen and gently raise the upper back, and head. Keep the feet and lower back flat on the floor. Exhale while pulling in the stomach, tighten the buttocks, and use the upper half of the back to lift 5 or 6 inches off the ground.

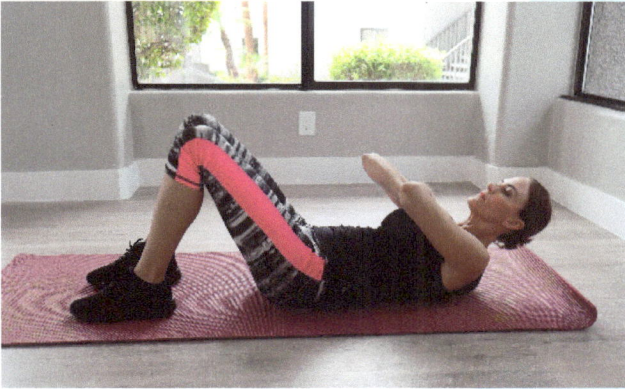

25. Situps for Lower Abdomen

Place hands behind the head and repeat the above to aid the lower abdomen.

Yummy for the tummy!

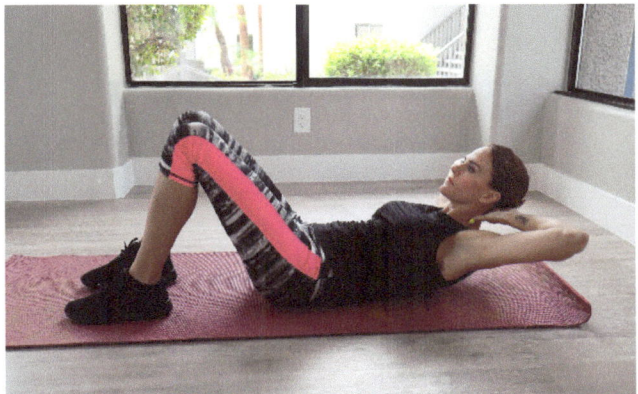

26. Side Leg Stretch

Lie flat on the back with knees bent. Keep the small of the back on the floor, Place arms against on the floor to the sides of the body. Bring the knee on one leg up the abdomen, stretch leg up, putting the heel towards the ceiling. Tighten buttocks. Exhale and slowly move the straight leg to the side with the heel towards the wall. Inhale and keep leg spread wide for a few moments.
Bring the leg straight up again where the heel is facing the ceiling, bend the knee, relax the buttocks, and repeat. The Side Leg Stretch is a wonderful inner thigh stretch and helps to firm up the lower back!

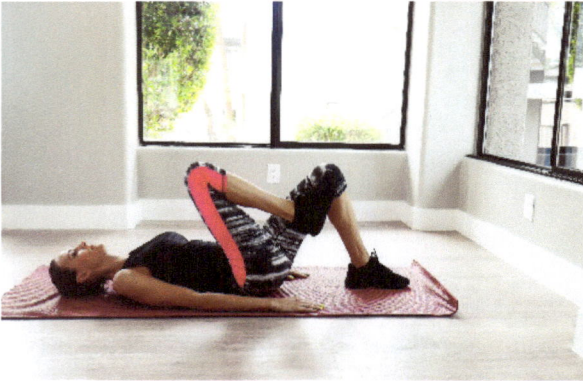

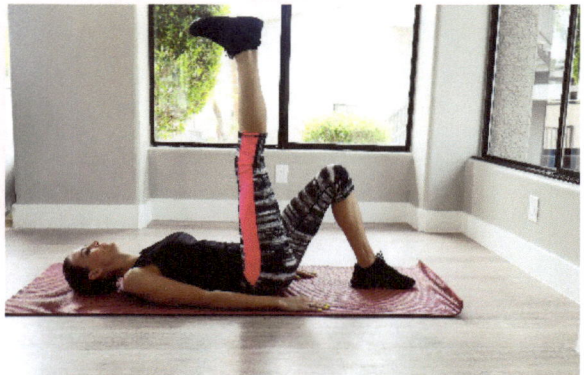

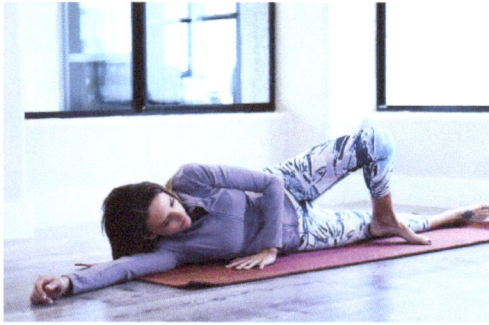

Safely Roll Onto Hands and Knees

To get up safely, place the arm straight above the head, use the other hand and the upper leg and foot to support the body as you roll up to the knees.

Tip: Be careful of the wrist to make sure they can handle the weight. If not, see the alternative on the next page.

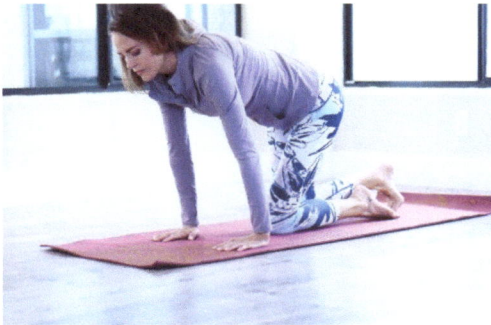

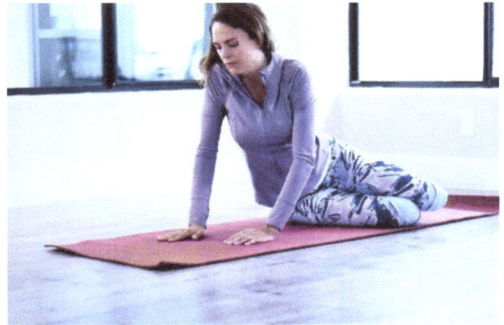

Happy body, better mind, and easier sleep.

27. Knee and Leg Raises

From a hands and knee, kneeling position. Lift the knee of one leg towards the chest. Stretch leg straight back with a pointed toe and tighten the buttocks. Lift and point to make the leg as long as possible. Repeat 10 counts for each side.

~~~~~~

Tip: Do not be tempted to do fast.
A slow, even speed will give the best results.

~~~~~~

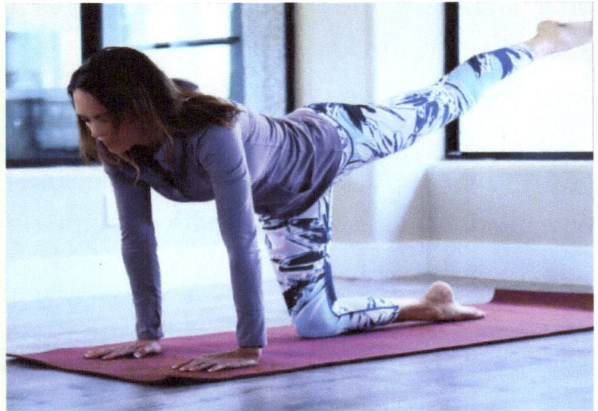

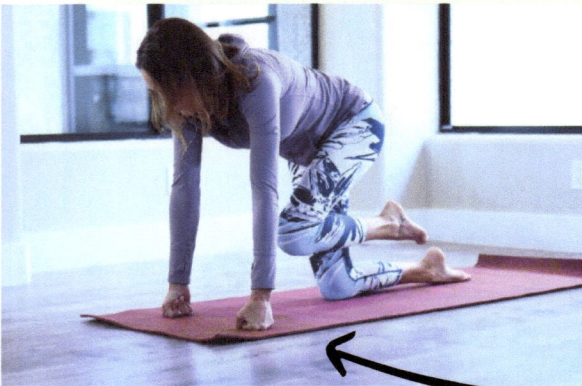

If you have wrist damage, then make a fist instead to help hold the weight. Face the knuckles as shown. Try not to arch the back.

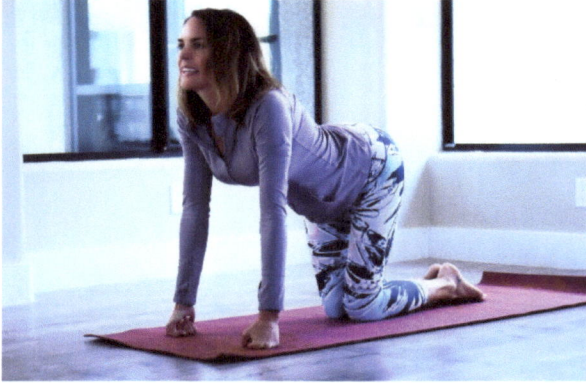

Let the head gently drop. Tuck the pelvic under and pull the navel towards the spine, and arch the back up towards the ceiling. Breathe deeply. Hold 15-30 seconds. Repeat.

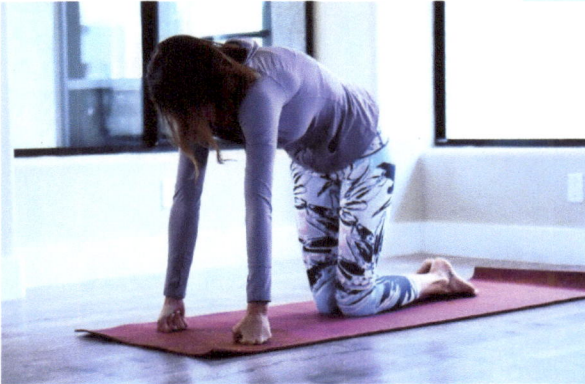

Meow!

28. Cat Stretch

On hands that are shoulder-width apart and knees are either together or hips-width apart. Pull shoulders away from the ears. Exhale, tighten the abdomen muscles and the buttocks. Lift the head tall and arch the lower back stretching it. Hold for 15-30 seconds

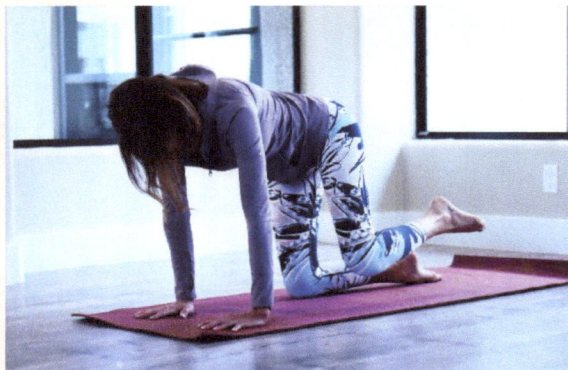

Talk about a bum-burn!

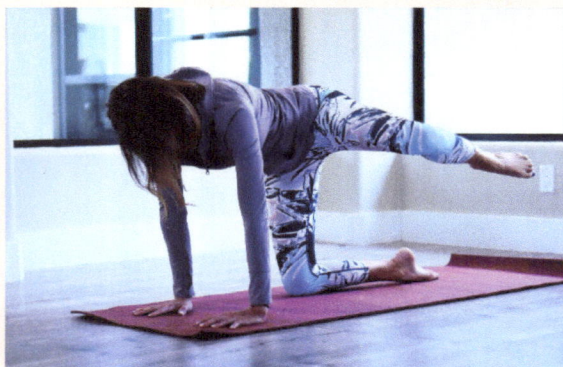

Sizzling

29. Doggie Leg Lifts

The leg is in an L shape throughout the exercise. Tighten the core of the body and slowly lift one leg without changing the L shape. Lift it away from the side of the body.

Keep the leg in an L shape. The head and spine aligned. Lift and lower for 10 repetitions and repeat on the other side. The knee should be an inch or so off the floor between lifts. Try not to move different parts of the body and keep hips as level as you can. Just lift the leg. So great for the bum!

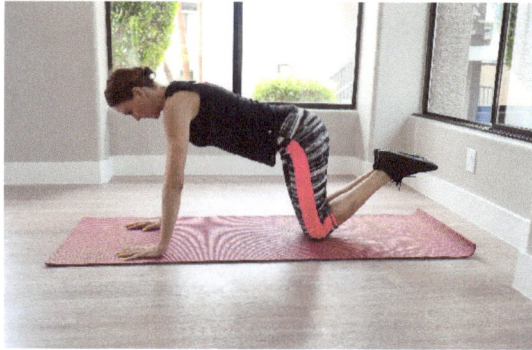

30. Push-Ups

Place either knuckles or palms on the floor, hands shoulder-width, arms straight with loose elbows, knees on the floor. Bend the elbows to bring nose close to the floor; rise and repeat. Do not arch the back. Add cushion to the knees if needed. Even a folded towel can make a difference.

Tip: There are many ways to do push-ups. ***Proper form is an absolute must!*** Push-ups are one of the best exercises for overall body toning and strengthening.

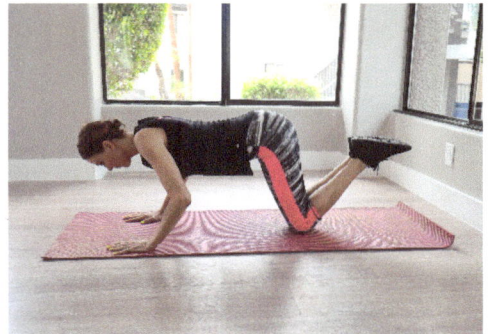

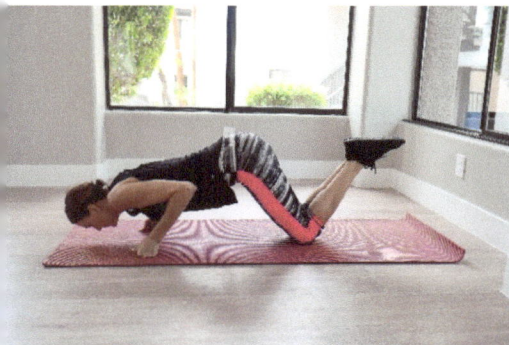

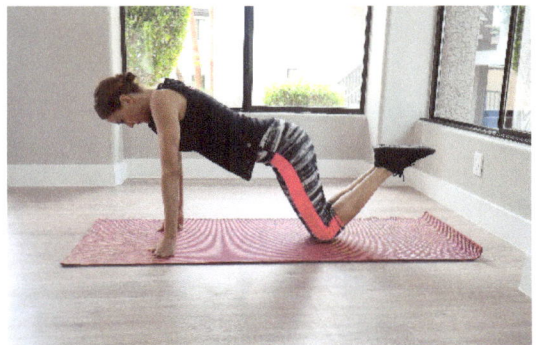

31. Stand Up and Stand Tall

Get up carefully, making sure the body is stable and supported while rising.

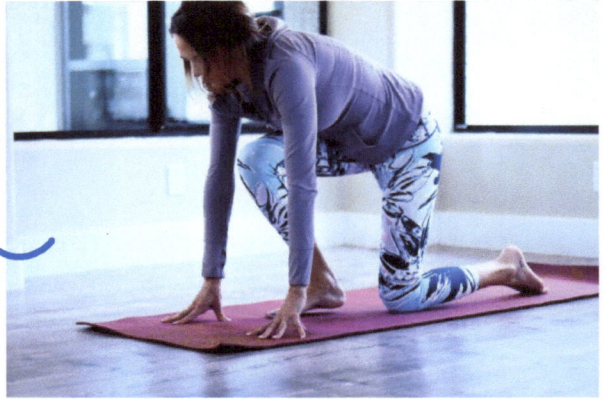

Picture toxins being released; yes, please!

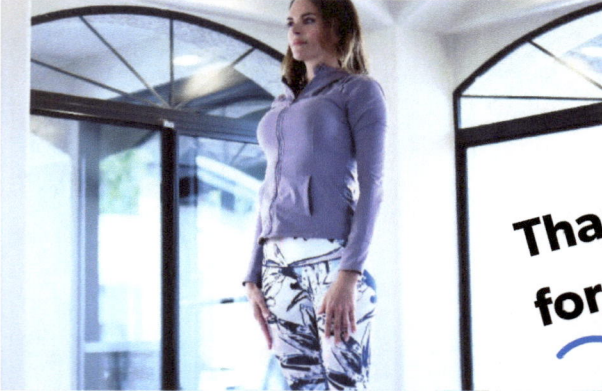

Thank you, body, for supporting me!

Stand up tall with the spine aligned straight, slightly relax the knees. Slightly tuck pelvic under and forward. Breathe deeply.

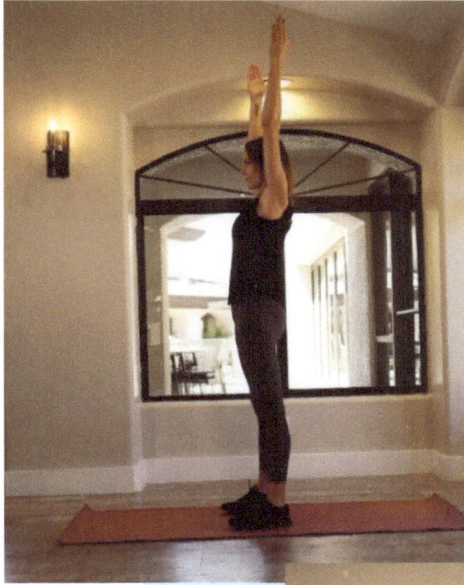

32. Standing Side Stretch

Stand tall with legs shoulder-width apart. Arms straight up with palms facing and shoulder width apart. Bend at the waist to one side, stretch the opposite side. Unbend and stand tall. Repeat on the other side. Excellent for aiding posture by strengthening the tissue around the ribs and spine.

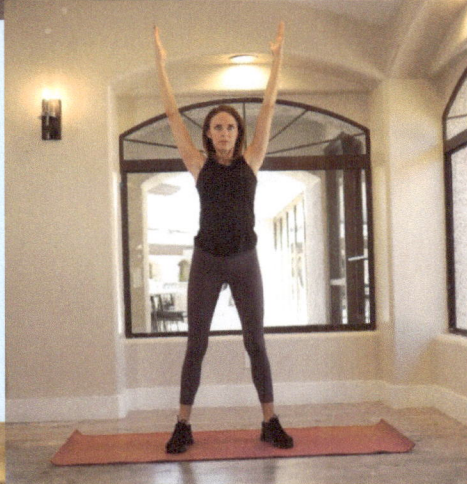

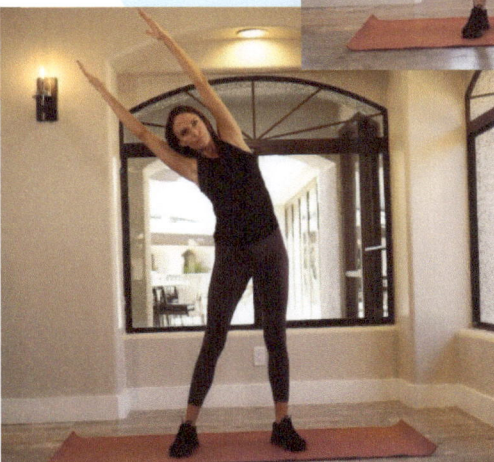

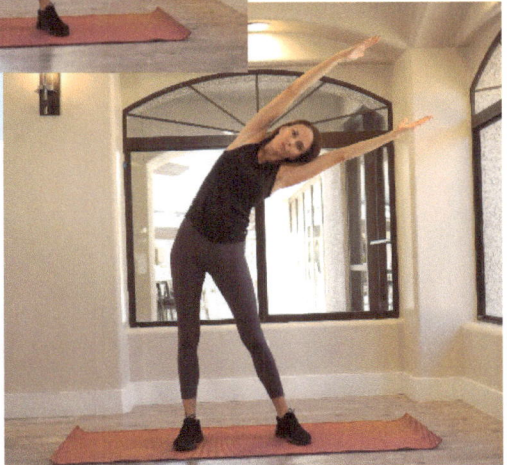

33. Ridding Negative Energy

Stand tall with the feet shoulder-width apart. Stretch arms out about chest high. Palms facing ground. Bend the elbows and bring the palms toward the pelvis, up the body, and then throw out the negative or sabotaging energy.

Get that crap out

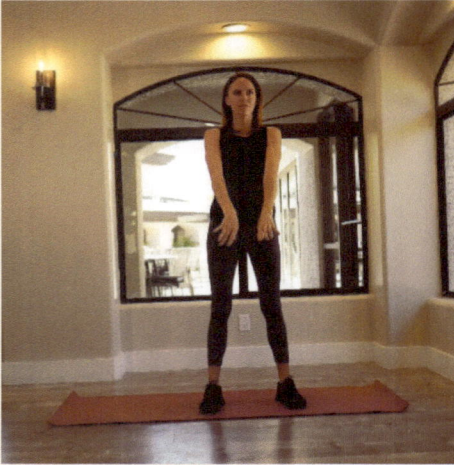

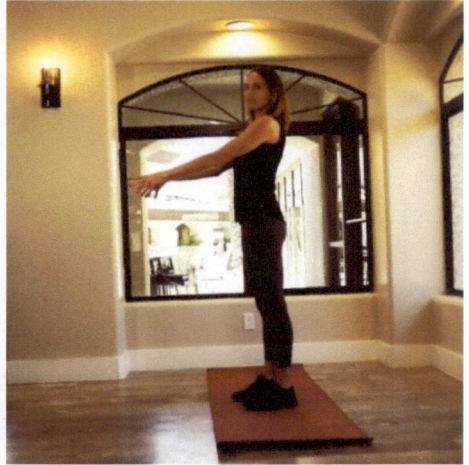

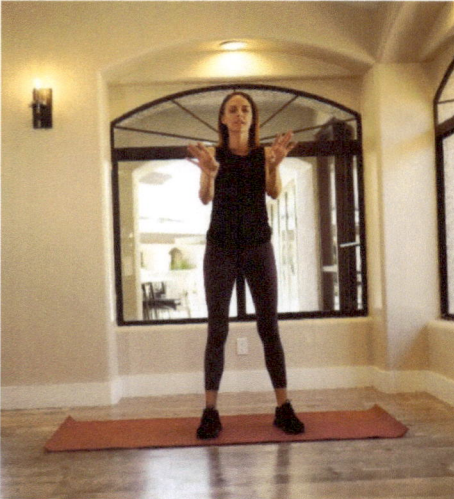

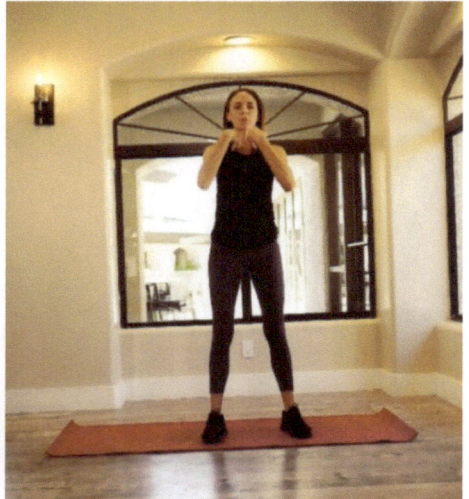

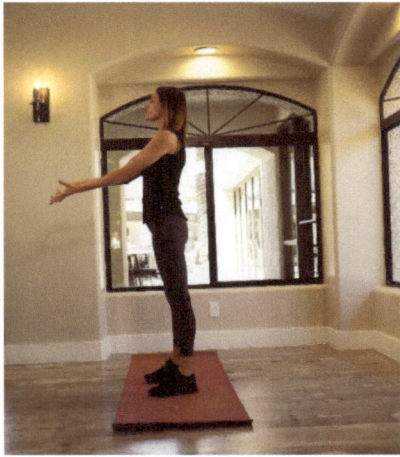

34. Stirring in the Positive Energy

Stand tall. Feet are shoulder-width apart. Place arms stomach high, out in front as if carrying several pieces of firewood. Palms are facing up. As if bringing in positive and loving energy. Bring hands towards chest and bring the positive energy in.

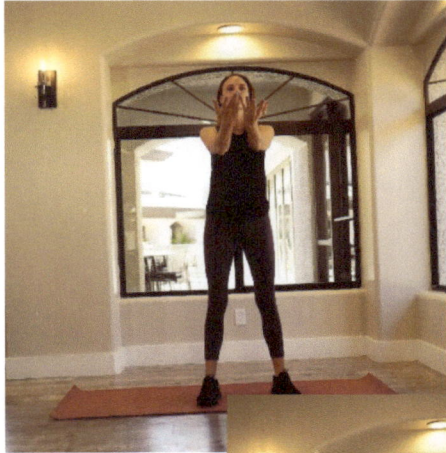

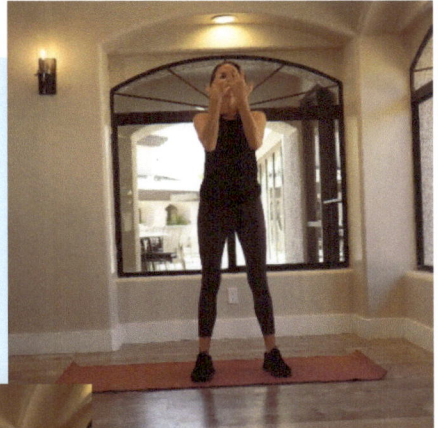

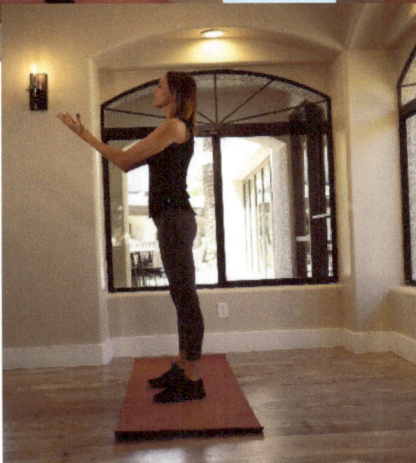

Pull The Love In!

35. Horse-Stance

Use a chair for support and to aid in proper posture. Hold on to the back of the chair. Point toes slightly out. Bend the knees and gently sit into the position. Hold this 15-30 seconds and repeat.

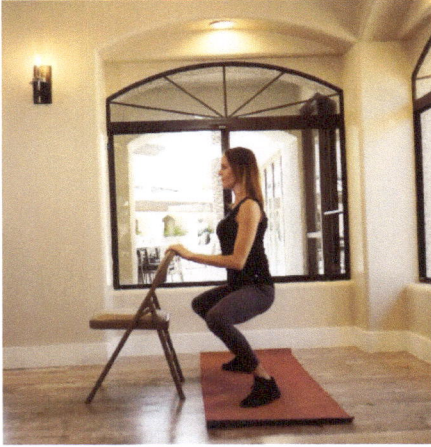

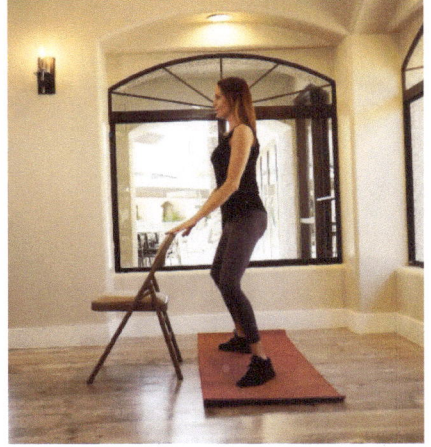

Tips: As the body gets stronger the chair. Can be removed. This is proper Horse Stance.

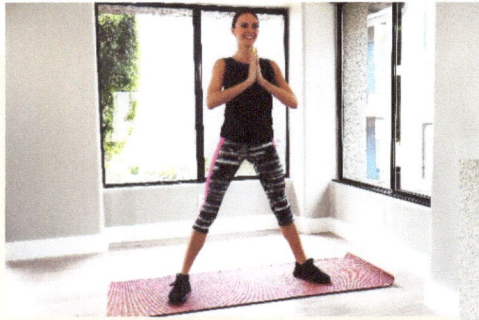

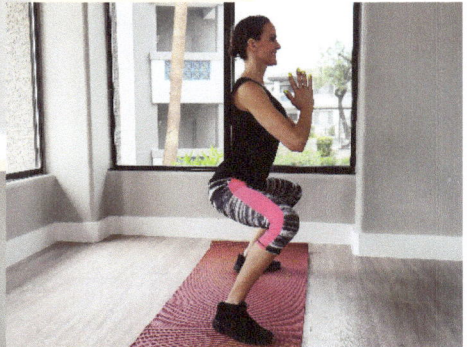

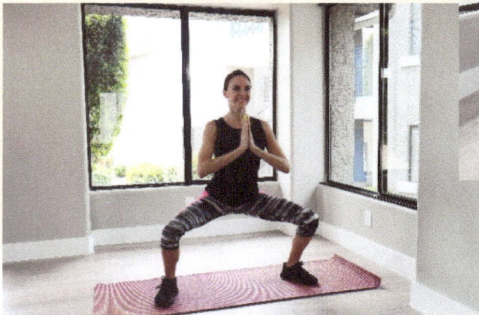

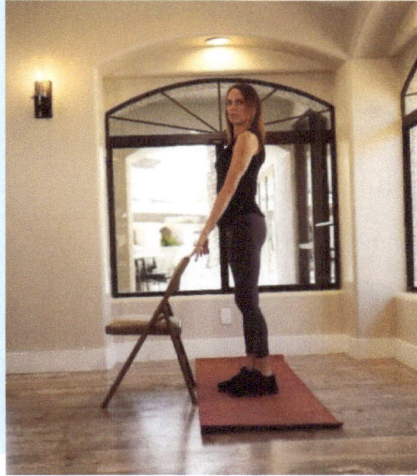

36. Calf Lift

Standing up tall, hold on lightly to the back of the chair. Legs should be hip-width. Bend the knee, lift the foot, and face the heel towards the back wall. Flex and point toes a few times. Press the foot back to stretch the leg. Bring knee and leg back, and place the foot on the floor. Repeat

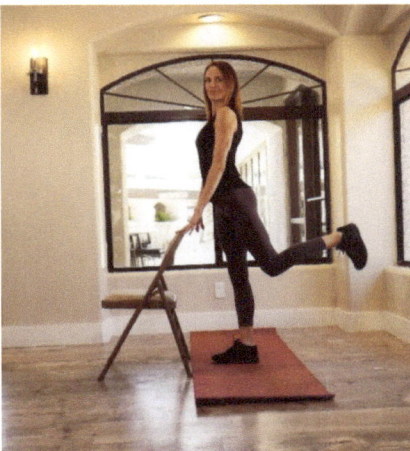
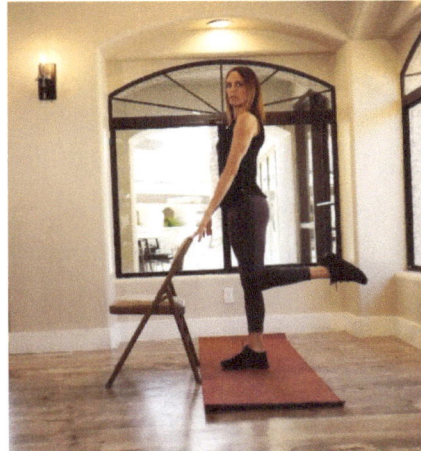

37. Side Chair Calf Lift

Stand to the side of the chair. Place hand on the chair back for balance. Keep body tall and still except for the leg exercising. Repeat the above calf lift

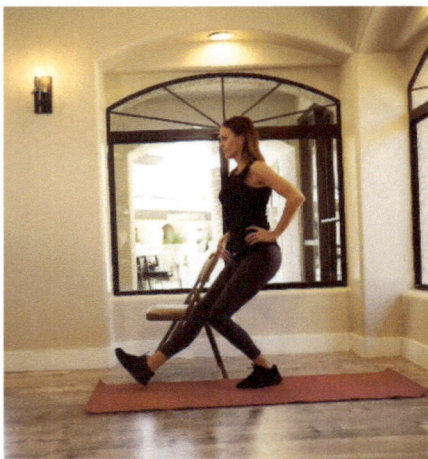
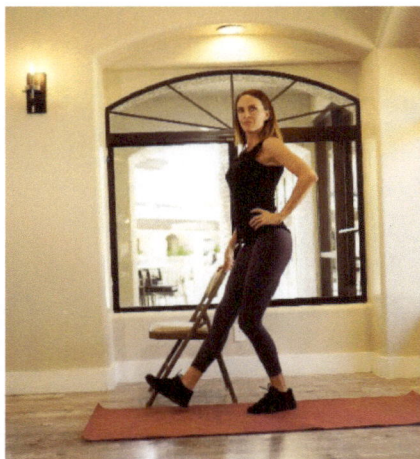

~~~~~~

38. Side Chair Calf Stretch

Stand tall next to chair. Hold on for balance. Stretch one leg out front, keeping foot flexed, and gently lower the upper body. The heel should touch the floor.
The lower you go, the bigger the stretch. Mild discomfort is okay, but pain is not. Rise back up to standing and repeat.

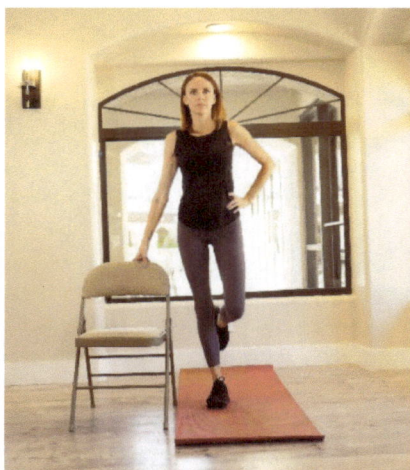

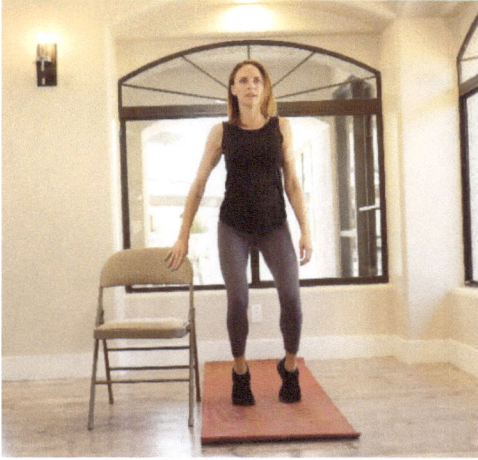

Oooh, what a stretch!

39. Plantar Fasciitis Stretch

Stand tall next to the chair with a hand on the back for balance. Spread the feet about hip-width. Rise up on the balls and toes. Slowly lower the buttocks and bend the knees as if sitting down part way. Keep the spine straight and tall.

Tips: The fasciitis ligament runs along the center bottom of the foot from the toes and attaches like slightly spread fingers to the heel. This exercise stretches it to help keep it flexible, strong, and from shrinking.

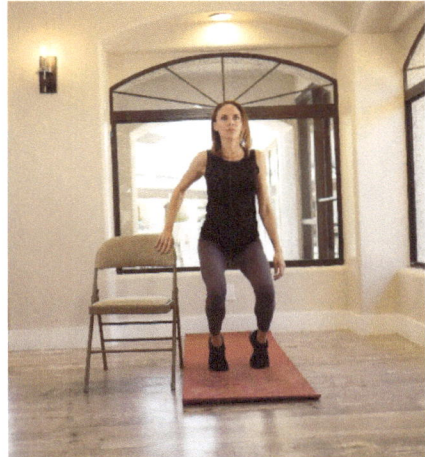

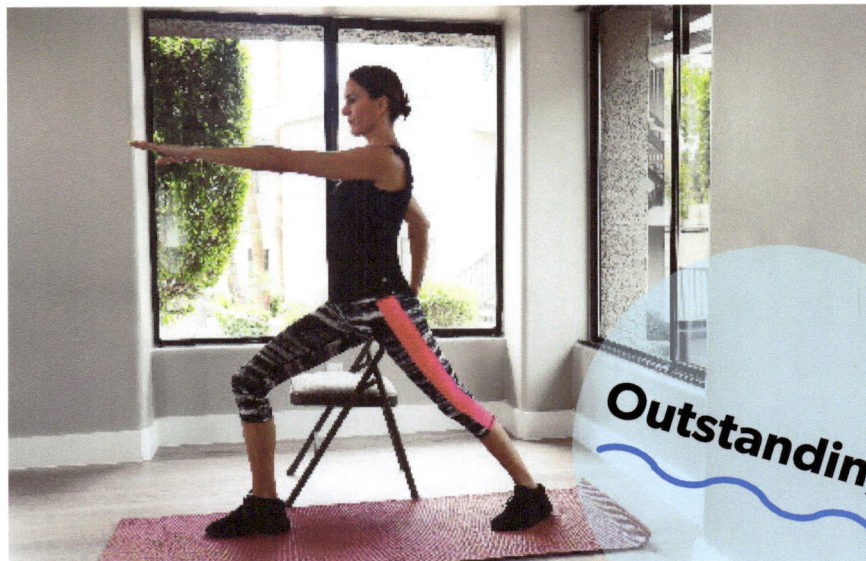

Outstanding!!!

40. Lunge with Straight Leg

Stand tall next to a sturdy chair with hand on the chair back.
Keep spine tall, head square to the shoulders, and hips lined
up with spine. Lift and extend the opposite arm from the chair,
and point fingers and arm straight out in front of the body.
Step forward with one leg. Bend the front knee as shown in
the picture. Keep the foot directly below the knee and the
back straight. Turn the back-leg foot slightly out for better
balance. Lower the body into a lung and hold 15-30 seconds.

I choose feeling great!

Tips: To increase the stretch and use different muscles, bend
the back knee, and widen the stance. Lunges strengthen the
hamstring and quadriceps.

41. Sitting Leg and Knee Stretches

Sit tall and straight in the chair. Put one ankle on top of the leg lower thigh. Gently place hand on the knee and add a little pressure to stretch.

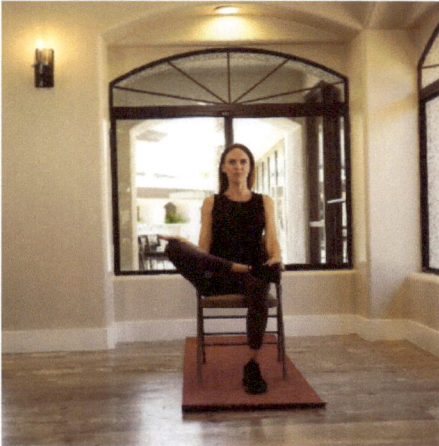
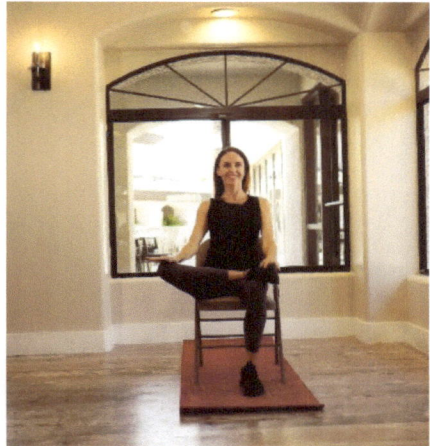

42. Knee Circles

Sit tall. Support the back of the thigh with the hands.
Lift the knee and slowly do large circles.

SMILE – it changes disruptive energy!

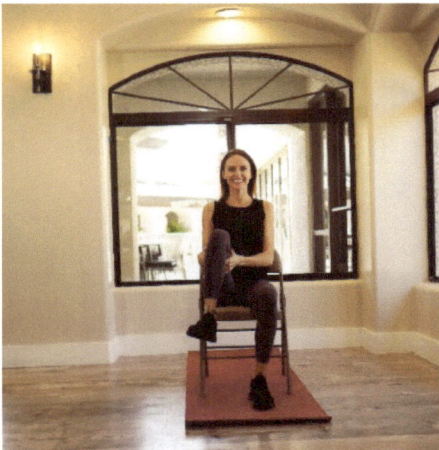
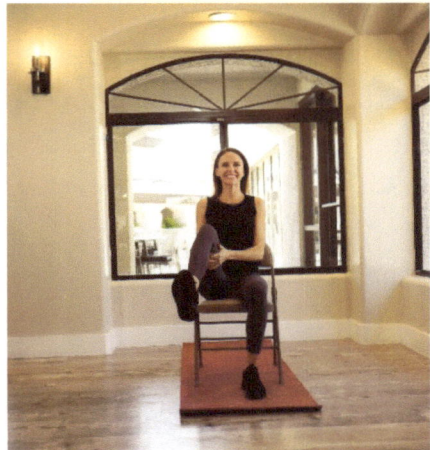

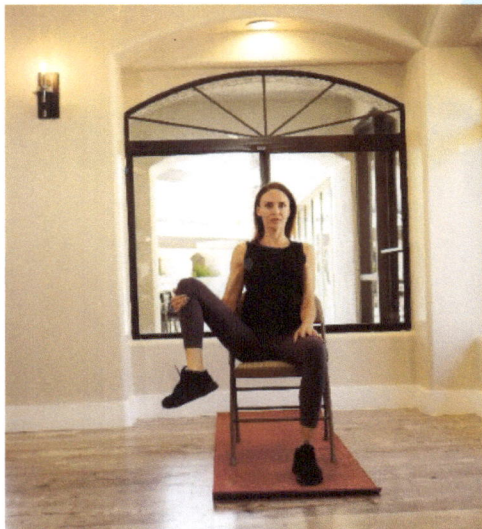

Keeping the hips swaying!

43. Sitting Knee and Thigh Stretch

Sit tall. Feet flat on the floor. Raise one leg, support under the knee, and pull to the side of the body as shown. Hold for 15-30 seconds. Repeat

💕 **The final following exercise is my absolute most favorite.** It is the Wuji used in Qi Gong.

Definition: Qi Gong (chi koon) is an ancient (960-1279 CE) Chinese art of moving energy. It is a practice in aligning breath, movement, and awareness for aiding and balancing health. It incorporates many arts such as: Confucianism, Taoism, Buddhism, traditional Chinese medicine and martial arts. Originally, the Wuji meant "ultimate", but now it is more like "primordial universe."

*I am supporting my body by moving so it can better support me! The body thinks and has its own brain, talk with it. Tell it that you are changing and it is not to draw you back but to support you in these healthy new habits. **Moving is simply joyful!**

Feeling Awesome!

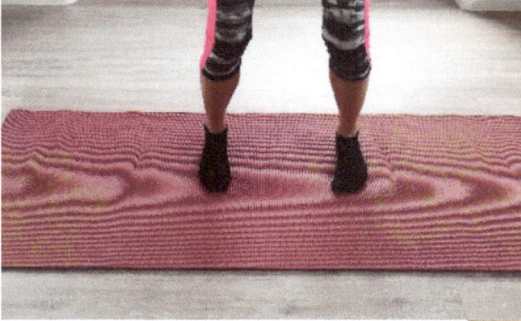

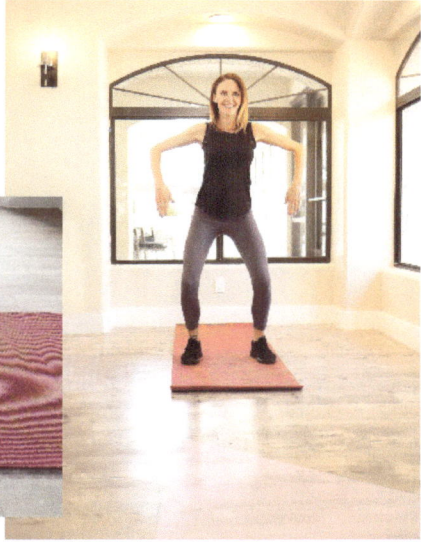

44. The Wuji (woo gee)

Stand tall. Keep the spine straight and pelvic slightly tucked forward, feet are shoulder-width, and slightly turned inward. Knees are flexed and relaxed. Bring the arms up bending the elbow, facing the fingers towards the earth, with palms facing the wall behind. Hold stance for 5-10 minutes to start. Take a cleansing breath. **Keep smiling!**

The Wuji is my most favorite of all the stances. One can hold this stance for a long period of time. I always end with this one!

*When done correctly, it is comfortable, steady, and relaxed. I picture myself like a human tree where the fingers go deep down into the supportive earth. I choose to connect to the heavens with a silver-blue ribbon. It starts from the heavens. Travels through the top of the head, and past the feet to connect to both the Divine and earth.

Clear the mind and notice any thoughts that flow through it. Notice them, and move them along.

Author Note:

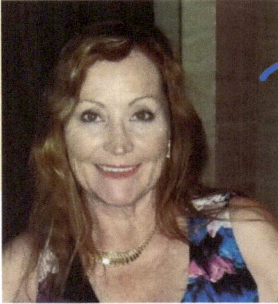

I was very active in a variety of sports, both for fun and competition. Even refereed and judged a season with basketball, gymnastics, and volleyball.

By the age of 47, I had been in two car accidents, had a work injury, sports damage, and essential life wear and tear on the body, which caused years of alternative approaches, medical treatments, and years of physical therapy. Nearly two decades of intense self and formal education, a slew of people guiding, teaching, and mentoring. It has helped me develop a unique set of skills to stay healthy and keep moving.

This is a personal battle; because I must for my quality of life, without movement it is greatly dampened. Losing this ability is not an option. One way or another keep moving! The Universe is a most fascinating and mystical place. I firmly believe we can regain health at every level. Love to learn and strive to be a good representation of humanity.

These pages contain my go-to routine. It is a blessing beyond measure to share this. I hope it makes exercise fun, healing, and freeing.

Divine love. Thank you, *Sherry*

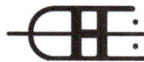

Holistic Collaboration Series Presents Book #2

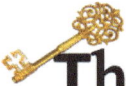

The Movement Connection

An Adaptable Exercise Routine for Flexibility and Strengthening

Body and Soul Nutrition

Sherry Bainbridge PhD, is an Author, Naturopath, Hypnotherapist, Intuitive, and Reiki Master. She is studied in Eastern, Tribal, and Western health/spiritual phylosophies.

https://holisticcollaboration.com
holisticcollaboration@gmail.com

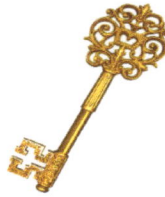

There are many vital keys to learning how to rid resistance towards healing the thoughts and actions that can hold us back. These keys open doors to eventually learning how to listen, influence, and create a fabulous life with wisdom and peace in a chaotic and multi-manipulating world. This is more than just a routine. It is intended to enliven the body, the mind, and the spirit. This type of guidance is necessary in reaching a higher and more nurturing state-of-being. Where beliefs are intentionally combined with strong, passionate feelings to positively influence present and future thinking, actions, reactions, and events.

When energy improves how we think and what feelings are attached to thoughts and then manifests through the physical. This routine is an opportunity to align the energy with the mind and the body. Always focusing within the space of gratefulness and healthy intentions for; healing, relaxing, prayer, or maybe just quieting the mind to observe what the sensations are saying.

Within us is the creator – the divine spark of life that connects us to many forms of communication and guidance.

The physical body has limitations that must be respected. Let go of resistance, smile, and kick it in the face. This is your body and your life, respect it! Start right here, right where you are, start, and don't look back. Movement is a precious gift to embrace! Ill health is profitable, stand up against the costly loss of movement. Support the body and work with it. Refuse to fall for any thinking that does not support this concept.

The more that join in on this type of self-care, the more light begins to brighten darkness in its many forms. Let's genuinely defy negative influences by treating others and ourselves with love, helpfulness, and compassion. There are physical and energetic laws. Each individual has power to change the future for not just themselves, but humanity as a whole. It starts with the individual, then it expands. Let's let the light of health shine and keep moving! You in?

Divine love, *Sherry*

www.ingramcontent.com/pod-product-compliance
Lightning Source LLC
Chambersburg PA
CBHW041225270326
41934CB00001B/4